Economists and Health Care

Economists and Health Care
From Reform to Relativism

Daniel M. Fox

PRODIST

New York • 1979

First Published in the United States of America
by PRODIST, a division of Neale Watson Academic Publications, Inc.
156 Fifth Avenue, New York, N.Y. 10010

Major portions of this book first appeared in the
Milbank Memorial Fund Quarterly,
David P. Willis, Editor.

©Milbank Memorial Fund Quarterly 1979

Additional materials
©Neale Watson Academic Publications, Inc. 1979

Library of Congress Cataloging in Publication Data

Fox, Daniel M
    Economists and health care.

    Includes commentaries.
    Bibliography: p.
    Includes index.
    1. Medical economics--History--20th century.
I. Title.
RA410.F69   338.4'7'36210904   79-22036
ISBN 0-88202-128-1

                Manufactured in the U.S.A.

CONTENTS

Foreword

DAVID P. WILLIS

ABOUT A YEAR AND A HALF AGO, a group of distinguished scholars was convened to discuss "Adequate Minimum Standards for Personal Health Services." Participants in the round table came from a wide range of academic, clinical, administrative, and political fields. A number of the prepared papers were illuminating, and have since been published in the *Milbank Memorial Fund Quarterly;* others were most informative for the ensuing discussion. Above all, perhaps, the conference proved to be instructive about the obstacles the conveners faced in realizing their hopes of creating a new way to formulate the questions about adequate minimum standards. This was to be prelude to yet a higher-level organizing concept, a more enlightened way to postulate resolutions.

The difficulties and disappointments of the undertaking might have been predicted:

> There is a wide gap between multi-disciplinary teams and inter-disciplinary teams. Multi-disciplinary applies when various disciplines provide their views with minimal cooperative interaction. Interdisciplinarity requires coordination among disciplines and synthesis of material through a higher-level organizing concept. . . . A good test of interdisciplinarity is whether a team can integrate imaginative ideas originating from different disciplinary perspectives so that the work product reflects an expanded lens of perception of reality. (Arnstein and Christakis, 1975: 159–160)

Edwin Newman, whose "civil tongue" is his personal amulet against linguistic miasmas, suspected pomposity here. I think he was wrong; imaginative ideas originating from different disciplinary perspectives can be pursued even while "strictly speaking." This book, much of which was originally published in the *Quarterly,* attempts to cut across a variety of traditional institutional and behavioral barriers. In exploring "economists and health care," diverse assumptions and divergent value systems have been drawn upon: history, economics, sociology, and political science. Most striking is the lack of any consistent *Weltanschauungen* (please note the Germanic precision, Mr. Newman) *within* the respective disciplines. Perhaps this should not have been so surprising. Note the following entry under "Sociology" in a turn-of-the-century encyclopedia:

> An unexact branch of economics. A hybrid invented by Comte to designate what was and is still known as social science, and was by the Greeks called politics. . . . [I]t would be premature [to regard it as] a science of human society or of man in his social and political relations. A vague and indeterminate study of that which scientists have not yet found to treat scientifically. In all, sociology would be of dwindling importance as a science compared with economics or anthropology. *(Nelson's Encyclopedia,* 1908)

Economists who are central to these discussions are not an unreasonably contentious lot resisting territorial incursions by a historian. Readers may recall the strictures set forth by the usually mild-mannered Francis D. Moore, M.D., against economists who engaged in medical subjects without having suitable prior medical training *(Milbank Memorial Fund Quarterly,* 1977). A number of communications from economists to the Editor expressed concern about implied professional insularity and intellectual isolationism. The challenge is now redirected!

Most contemporary scholars identified by Dr. Fox were invited to contribute commentaries on an earlier version of his essay, with special reference to the twin historical sins of omission and revisionism with respect to their own work. Professors Milton Friedman, Martin Feldstein, Victor Fuchs, and Selma Mushkin graciously declined with the resoluteness of Bartelby the scrivener. Their absence is regretted, most poignantly that of the doyenne of medical economists. Professor John Dunlop contributed through direct correspondence with Dr. Fox. Although none of the commentators attempted an *apologia pro sua vita,* each has given a disarming glimpse into highly personal and professional views and styles.

The comments are arranged solely to reflect one judgment of the nature of these differences. The reader may elect other orderings with equal profit and an expanded "perception of reality."

References

Arnstein, S. R., and Christakis, A. N. 1975. *Perspectives on Technology Assessment.* Jerusalem: Science and Technology Publishers.

Moore, F. D. 1977. Board Requirements for Economists Who Write on Medical Subjects? A Comment on *The Condition of Surgery. Milbank Memorial Fund Quarterly/Health and Society* 55 (Fall): 455–460.

Nelson's Encyclopedia. 1908. London: Thomas Nelson.

Preface

Of Economists and Economics, Ceteris Paribus

GERALD ROSENTHAL

National Center for Health Services Research,
Department of Health, Education, and Welfare

THE PAPER BY PROFESSOR FOX examines the role and influence of economists and economics (not the same thing) on the public discussion of health policy in the United States by examining the economics literature. Kenneth Boulding once defined economics as "what economists do!" Nevertheless, economics, like other academic disciplines, tends to regard some activities as more "legitimate" than others. While the particular activities that are revered may change over time, the source of legitimization remains the academic setting; and the models that guide the interests and careers of the newly "ordained" are the professors who have achieved academic success by publishing in academic journals and contributing to the knowledge base of the discipline. It is not inappropriate, therefore, for an historian to attempt to identify the nature of the interest in health care issues of economists by examining the published articles in the major journals of the field. This investigation has led Professor Fox to conclude that the earlier interest in reform on the part of economists has been submerged and replaced by an interest primarily directed at methodological applications and "fine tuning."

As evidenced by the accompanying papers, response to this conclusion varies considerably among a group of individuals, all of whom have been, and remain, participants in this experience. I. S. Falk, the most "reform-minded" (there is no pejoration implied), argues that the early work was more "legitimate" economics by economists than Fox gives credit for. Kenneth Arrow, the most disciplinarily "legitimate" (again, not a pejorative), argues that the contemporary selection of topics reflects "reform" considerations. For most of us, Fox's paper provides one additional perspective on the rather complex relation between the value of economics and the values of economists. To the extent that it can contribute to a further understanding of both the utility and the limits of economic analysis as a component of the public policy process, we can all benefit.

In the past decade or so, economists have given lawyers a good run for the title "most numerous professional group in Washington." Every proposed new piece of legislation is accompanied by economic analyses from both supporters and opponents. Since economists are part of the process of policy development and implementation, it is important for us to understand what they can and cannot bring to that process *as economists*.

The interest of economists in issues of health and welfare dates from the first economist. The pursuit of that interest is what stimulated the development of economics and the learning of economics, not the other way around. Nevertheless, as the discipline formed, the conflict between narrowing inquiry to obtain analytic power and the pursuit of understanding of the total problem has characterized the field.

Perhaps the maximum commitment to the latter is represented by the peculiarly American institutionalist school of economics. Economists like Ely and Commons aggressively pursued reforms in labor law, income security, and health policy. Discussions of these issues were important components of labor economics texts of the twenties and thirties. The commitment to dealing with economic issues in the context of their institutional realities influenced many of the labor economists. They regarded the process of collective bargaining as being as important to understanding and determining the wage rate as is knowledge of the supply and demand curve for labor.

Institutional economists have a history of involvement in the policy process at both the state and federal levels. The tradition continues in Wisconsin, where the most recent director of the state health department was a professor of economics on leave. In earlier days, the institutionalists were also well accepted as part of the "legitimate" corps of economists. They were leaders in many strong departments of economics and held high office in the associations of the discipline.

In those days, the notion that mainstream economics (as opposed to economists) was not interested in reform would have been invalid on its face. Today, notwithstanding the ever greater involvement of economists in the policy process, that assertion can find much support. An examination of the factors that might account for the change in perception and, perhaps, in reality, is clearly in order and Professor Fox's paper provides a useful and needed stimulus for this inquiry.

To some extent, this perception reflects the development of economics from the moral philosophy of the past to the highly analytic quantitative exercise typical of contemporary applications. Economics, as do all social sciences, attempts to focus on only certain aspects of human behavior. By limiting the scope of inquiry, it is possible to develop more informative analyses. In simple terms, we increase the power of analysis by leaving out some of the complexity. Because economics deals with aspects of human behavior that appear to display great consistency in their "pure" form, we economists have developed more extensive theory and more powerful analyses than have other social scientists. To the complex problems of human existence the economist brings order, analytic power, and specific quantitative answers. He does this by leaving out many variables for which we have no consistent theory. The seductiveness of the rationality of *ceteris paribus* is hard to overestimate.

It is to the development and refinement of these precise quantitative tools and the development of theoretical underpinnings that the discipline has directed its major attention over the past few decades. The field honors those who contribute to this end and publishes in its journals the record of their work. Little wonder, then, that the published literature of the "mainstream" in economics seems devoid of prescription for reform. By limiting analysis to the orderly and quantifiable, we deliberately omit many considerations that contribute to a solution for most consequential problems. *Ceteris paribus* determines what we investigate rather than how we interpret. We have forsaken breadth of issue for power of analysis.

If the emphasis noted by Fox on "relativism" rather than "reform" reflects the development of economics, how are we to account for the expanding involvement of economists in the policy-making process as well as in the management of government programs within the health area? If the *field* rewards quantitative analysis and the development of theory, how do we account for the growth in the numbers of trained economists turning their attention to problems in health and medical care from the mid-1960s to the present?

Three distinct circumstances probably contribute. First, the application of economic analytic techniques proved to be a powerful addition to decision making in the Department of Defense in the early 1960s. Problems often could be bounded by strategic considerations. This made *ceteris paribus* a much less restrictive assumption than is the case in many other areas of decision making. It also provided a framework for quantification of choices, a process that allowed the analysis to select the policy from a set of alternatives derived from other sources. This provided great impetus to acceptance of the economist as partner in the policy process without requiring him to compromise his analytic integrity to policy considerations. By the mid-1960s, all federal agencies were attempting to exploit the power of economic analysis on behalf of program objectives. This clearly created a market for those with economic training, without regard to expertise in the area of application.

A second influence was the increased awareness, stimulated by Medicare and Medicaid, of the large and growing economic resources being devoted to the production and distribution of medical care services. The sheer size of the sector attracted the attention of economists, both in the academic setting and in high positions in policy circles such as the Council of Economic Advisors and the Joint Economic Committee of the Congress. Growing public and political awareness of the relevance of notions of scarcity, opportunity cost, trade-offs, and efficiency to discussions of health policy provided additional opportunity to incorporate the language and analytic strategies of the economist into the public decision-making process.

A third influence reflects the development in economics of more complex and elaborate theories of economic behavior potentially susceptible to empirical testing and refinement. More and more of the literature of economics was devoted to the results of such testing. The emphasis on quantitative analysis increased the dependency of economists on the availability of data. The burgeoning medical care sector had two attributes that made it an appealing locus for the work of young economists. First, it generated considerable amounts of data as a result of the elaborate record keeping inherent in the nature of medical practice, on the one hand, and growing public financing and regulation, on the other. Second, much contemporary economic theory had not been generalized to the nonprofit sector of the economy and the growing interest in medical care provided an environment susceptible to such testing. For the young economist seeking to establish a reputation by research and publication, the application of accepted theory to a new sector of the economy that could provide sufficient data for complex econometric analysis proved an almost irresistible attraction. For many, it was the application of the tools of economic analysis and not the substance of the field of application that accounted for the attention.

In the past five or six years, new trends have been emerging. Although not explicitly addressed in Professor Fox's paper, these changes may have significance for the interpretation we give to Fox's observations. First, a growing number of economists are pursuing career paths not primarily situated within traditional academic departments. Professional schools (of medicine as well as of public health, administration, etc.), training the manpower of the health care industry, are becoming hospitable environments for the academic careers of economists interested in health care. The trend toward joint appointments for economists primarily situated in the professional school continues, providing linkage to the discipline while enhancing institutional influence on the research undertaken and the preferred outlets for publication. The volume of economics papers appearing in journals dealing with medical care, health services research, and administration gives some indication that, for many young economists, significant changes are taking place in the traditional paths to professional success, even within an academic career.

A second influence, particularly among health economists, is a growing tendency to consider some public experience at the federal, state, or local level as a natural part of the professional economist's experience. Many of these jobs involve considerable decision making and, as such, provide settings within which both the power and the limits of economic analysis are evidenced daily. That lesson is a telling one and affects every economist who has that experience in the health care field. As such individuals return to the academic setting, the teaching of health economics should itself be affected. This has been true of *labor economics* for many years and is beginning to

influence the younger field of *health economics* in much the same
way.

While such changes may not immediately affect what
economics can do, they are likely to change significantly what
economists do! To the extent that Professor Fox's paper points out
the difference between our professional public face and reality, we
can be grateful for the lesson. To the extent that our reality is not
what we think it is, more than gratitude is needed for an adequate
response. Professor Fox's paper and the responses to it provide a
beginning for understanding.

From Reform to Relativism:
A History of Economists
and Health Care

DANIEL M. FOX

Health Sciences Center,
State University of New York at Stony Brook

SIGNIFICANT CHANGES HAVE OCCURRED during the past thirty years in the assumptions made by social scientists and particularly by economists interested in the organization and financing of health services. Social scientists who studied health and medical care earlier in the century were primarily concerned with promoting measures to reduce the financial burden of illness on individuals and families and to make services more accessible. In the past thirty years, scholars have increasingly separated their research, for which they claim objectivity, from their commitments on disputed public issues. Like other social scientists, health services researchers have exchanged advocacy for neutrality during the past generation. As a result of this exchange, social scientists who work on health issues have become both more respected within their disciplines and more acceptable to physicians but less openly concerned with equity and social justice.

This paper explores the changing assumptions of social scientists concerned with health services and medical care, by surveying the history of attention given to these subjects by professional economists in the United States during the past century. Most professional economists in this century have worked in colleges and universities; but many of them have been employed by government agencies, voluntary associations, research organizations, and, in a few cases, professional associations and pressure groups. The word "economist" in this paper is defined narrowly, to mean men and women with advanced academic training in economics who apply the theory and methods of the discipline in their work. The reasons for using this definition are explained and the sources used in research are described in the "Note on Methods and Sources" at the end of the paper.

A major theme of this paper is the uneasy relationship or tension between advocacy and objectivity as purposes for research in economics. Economists throughout the history of the discipline have espoused both purposes. What is examined here is not the desirability of one or the other purpose but rather the gradual change in economists' views of their starting assumptions in approaching the health sector of the economy and the link between these assumptions and their research. For roughly the first half of this century, most economists who studied health affairs assumed that most citizens needed more medical care. That is, they assumed that health services were, in general, beneficial and in insufficient supply. These assumptions made most of them advocates of compulsory health insurance and gradual reform to increase access to services.

Since the 1950s, economists studying health services and medical care have increasingly focused their research on questions about the allocation of resources to and within the health sector. They have generally not infused their work with strong convictions about the worth of these resources. Research that analyzes alternative ways to allocate resources produces a kind of economic literature different from that based on the premise that resources are insufficient, badly distributed, or both. This difference, and why it developed, is the principal theme of this paper. As an aid to communication, when arraying data and presenting my argument I shall refer to this gradual change in the purposes of economists' research as the difference between reform and relativism as professional stances.

The social sciences have become increasingly specialized in the past century. In the last third of the nineteenth century, American scholars who were trained in Germany, or according to German models, developed the modern disciplines of economics, sociology, and political science. By the first decade of the twentieth century, these disciplines had replaced moral philosophy or vaguely defined social science as the basis for organizing academic departments, journals, and professional associations. German models of academic organization persisted in the twentieth century, despite the decline of German influence on work in the social sciences and especially in economics. Although the intellectual connections among members of the various disciplines were closer at the turn of the century than they are today, the trend toward increased specialization within the discipline was clear to contemporary observers. Within each of the disciplines, moreover, a tension between science and the advocacy of social reform was acknowledged early in the century.

The increasing specialization of social scientists, and of economists in particular, contrasts sharply with the broad subject matter physicians have associated with the term "medical economics." During this century, medical economics has meant such activities as gathering financial and social information about recipients of medical services, making more efficient the financing and administration of hospitals, promoting public and voluntary health insurance, describing the health problems of industry and labor and, perhaps most important, the proper conduct of the business aspects of the practice of medicine.

In the first half of this century, unlike the years since about 1960, there were few connections between the subjects called "medical economics" and the discipline of economics. A striking example in point is a survey of instruction in medical economics by medical colleges in the United States in 1937. At a time when professional economists were preoccupied with studies of business cycles and debating new theories of monopolistic competition and welfare economics, the following subjects were taught as "medical economics":

> Medical Ethics, Medical History, Public Health Administration and Relations, Medical Jurisprudence, Office Management, Cults and Quackery, Hygiene and Preventive Medicine, Relation of Physicians to Public, Psychiatry, Medical Insurance, Collections, Physician's Investments, Birth Control and Contraception, Abortion, Euthanasia, Eugenics, Pastoral Medicine, Hospital Appointments and Medical Journalism. (American Medical Association: 1937)

There are three distinct periods in the history of the relations between the disciplines of economics and medicine. Economics and medicine, though linked in intriguing ways in the seventeenth and eighteenth centuries, diverged in the nineteenth century. During the first two decades of the twentieth century, however, economists, both academics and activists with graduate training in economics, became increasingly involved in health affairs, particularly in the issue of compulsory insurance. This involvement was demonstrated in research, articles in professional journals and popular magazines, and service on committees organized by public agencies, pressure groups, and philanthropic organizations.

In the second period, from the 1920s until just after World War II, professional economists were in general uninterested in research and reform relating to medical care. This lack of interest was a result of forces both within and external to the discipline of economics.

In the third period, which began in the 1950s, economists became increasingly active in research on health care issues. The origins and results of this increased activity are far from clear. Contemporary history is a treacherous subject. Many people still active have strong opinions about their own and others' contributions.

Medicine and Economics Before the Twentieth Century

More extensive formal relations between medicine and what is now economics existed in the seventeenth and eighteenth centuries than at any subsequent time until the present. Several physicians made important contributions to the development of knowledge about the production, distribution, and consumption of wealth. John Locke's work in politics and the theory of knowledge was seminal in the history of the social sciences and needs to be understood in the context of his experience as a physician. William Petty in England and François Quesnay in France, both physicians, participated in the development of modern economic doctrines. Bernard Mandeville, a London physician of Dutch origin, has a significant place in the history of social analysis foreshadowing the elaboration of classical economic theory. These men brought to their work in economics a profound sense of the value of individual human effort and of the social costs of illness (Clark, 1971; Hutchinson, 1964; Mini, 1974; Routh, 1975).

From the middle of the eighteenth to the early twentieth century, however, physicians and economists seem to have been members of intellectual networks that were segregated from each other.

Although the classical economists, notably Malthus, Ricardo, and the Mills, were deeply concerned with issues of subsistence, health, and disease, their work appears to have aroused little interest in the medical profession. Even where relations should logically have been close, in movements to reform sanitation and protect the public's health in England and Germany, for example, there was little connection between medical and economic ideas (Fox, 1979).

The influence of the English Benthamites, or Utilitarians, on public health legislation in the first half of the nineteenth century is an exception to this generalization. Jeremy Bentham and several of his disciples, especially Edwin Chadwick, developed plans to reorganize public health and medical care and to regulate medical practice. Benthamite influence was considerable on the establishment of legislative and administrative standards for public health. For a century, Benthamite principles dominated arguments for an expanded public role in the prevention of illness and for compulsory health insurance in England and in the United States. Particularly in England, but also in the United States, thorough reports about the condition of the poor, including their health status and access to services, were prepared as a result of the convergence of the Benthamite and the German Historical Schools of research in economics (Cowen, 1969; Cullen, 1975; Halévy, 1955; Roberts, 1960).

Despite the achievements of the Utilitarians, the histories of the development of modern medicine and of social science in the United States at the end of the nineteenth century are strictly parallel. Several thousand Americans studied social science in German universities from the 1870s to the 1890s. Many of them later became the first professional economists, sociologists, psychologists, and political scientists in American universities. During the same years, approximately fifteen thousand Americans received German medical degrees. Connections that could have existed between physicians and social scientists, because both groups were heavily influenced by German models of thought and education, were infrequent. Social scientists and physicians formed few significant alliances despite their common educational experiences and their subsequent employment by the same universities. They remained distant from each other while simultaneously advocating analogous changes in higher education, against strong resistance from entrenched academic and community interests. At such institutions as The Johns Hopkins University, the University of Pennsylvania, the

University of Wisconsin, and Harvard University, physicians and members of the social science disciplines had similar but separate concerns at the end of the nineteenth century (Bonner, 1963; Dorfman, 1949; Fox, 1967; Haskell, 1977; Herbst, 1965; Veysey, 1965).

Although the causes of the separation of medicine and the social science disciplines in the United States when both developed their modern theories, methods, and organizational structures are not clear, the effects were a series of missed opportunities. Physicians, with scattered exceptions, were not aware of the increased interest among social scientists from different disciplines in the behavior of groups and cultures and of their growing neutrality toward competing solutions for social problems. Similarly, many social scientists missed the implications of the emergence of an ethics of effectiveness among physicians, and of the increasing uncertainty, particularly among biomedical scientists, about the ease with which new scientific knowledge could be translated into improved health (Burns, 1977).

The Early Twentieth Century:
Connections Begin

Although medicine and social science were, in general, segregated from each other, there were many promising connections early in the twentieth century. The number and variety of articles in medical journals on economic subjects increased steadily after the turn of the century. For the first time, physicians were citing economists' arguments when writing for each other about insurance and the relation of services to the standard of living of the population. Economists, writing in their own journals, were beginning to take note of the health industry. Moreover, economists and physicians concerned with social reform were connected through work in settlement houses, in campaigns to control tuberculosis, venereal disease, prostitution, and the use of alcohol, and in organizations pressing for public attention to eugenics, nutrition, child welfare, workmen's compensation, and social insurance.

Several well-known professional economists wrote about health issues affecting public policy; they included Richmond Mayo-Smith, Henry Seager, and Edwin R. A. Seligman of Columbia University, Richard T. Ely and John R. Commons of the University of Wisconsin, Henry Farnam and Irving Fisher of Yale University, and Simon Patten of the University of Pennsylvania. Other economists, many of them students of these men, employed by public agencies, voluntary associations, and pressure groups, also applied the theory and methods of economics to such problems as paying for medical care, health and ·safety in industry, and the value of public health and preventive measures.

Economists interested in labor questions were among the first to pay attention to problems of health. As early as 1886, Ely, who with Patten and Edmund James had just written what became the call for the American Economic Association, discussed the relations of wages and health in his book, *The Labor Movement in America.* Ely and others were concerned with industrial accidents and legislation to regulate working conditions and provide compensation to victims. Labor economists' interest in health issues continued; in 1920 for instance, Carleton H. Parker, in *The Casual Laborer and Other Essays,* described the contributions of psychology, eugenics, and mental hygiene to understanding labor unrest (Dunlop, 1979).

Patten advocated the application of theories derived from both the German Historical School and neoclassical welfare economics to problems of social policy and the quality of life. Three of his students, William H. Allen, Edward T. Devine, and Henry R. Seager, wrote a great deal about what a later generation would call health economics (Fox, 1967). Allen, for example, as an employee of the Bureau of Municipal Research in New York City, applied economists' concepts of expense to problems of hospital efficiency and explored the implications of Patten's theories about potential abundance for health services (Allen, 1907; 1909). Devine, an economist with a seminal administrative role in professional social work, discussed issues of public health and entitlement to services in numerous books and papers. Seager, a professor of economics at Columbia University, published an influential book, *Social Insurance,* in 1912.

Other economists were deeply involved in the campaign for compulsory health insurance in the second decade of the century. John R. Commons, like Seager, was active in the American Association for Labor Legislation, which publicized workers' health risks and their limited access to care and was a major vehicle for the advocacy of reform. Another activist in the movement for social insurance, I. M. Rubinow, a physician, had studied economics at

Columbia with Seligman. Rubinow, a brilliant analyst of economic statistics, made an important contribution to the study of real wages and wrote a notable series of articles on health insurance published in 1915 in the *Journal of Political Economy* (Lubove, 1968; Nelson, 1969; Numbers, 1978; Rubinow, 1914; 1916).

The best known economist concerned with health issues was Fisher of Yale. A pioneer in the application of mathematics to economic analysis, he actively promoted changes in the health behavior of citizens, and advocated reform in the health policies of corporations and government agencies. In 1907 he founded the Committee of One Hundred on National Health to press for the creation of a department of health in the federal government. Two years later, he was the principal author of the *Report on National Vitality* issued by the National Conservation Commission appointed by President Theodore Roosevelt. He created the Life Extension Institute to persuade insurance companies that health education and physical examinations for policy holders would reduce untimely deaths and hence raise profits. Physicians began to promote his view that "health pays" in medical journals. Fisher was president of the American Association for Labor Legislation during the campaign for compulsory health insurance from 1912 to 1918 (Fisher, 1956).

This promising involvement of economists in health affairs soon ended. By the early 1920s, organized medicine was considerably more wary both of proposals for social reform and of nonmedical intellectual influence than it had been a decade earlier. Medical aloofness was, in part, a cautious response to professional success. Medical prestige and income were rising, in large part as a result of apparent scientific progress, growing public confidence in physicians, the gradual elimination of competition between "regular" physicians, and members of the numerous medical "sects" that lingered from the nineteenth century, and a declining ratio of physicians relative to population.

Moreover, the controversy over efforts to legislate compulsory health insurance in various states after 1912 deeply scarred both physicians and social scientists who advocated social reform. Throughout the first decade and a half of the century, most medical leaders, including those in the American Medical Association, believed that compulsory health insurance should be supported because it was inevitable. Many physicians also believed it was desirable. But medical opposition to compulsory insurance increased and was organized to become politically effective in just a few years after 1912. As Ronald Numbers has recently argued, health insurance, under sharp attack by physicians who feared limitations on their ability to practice freely and on their incomes, suffered a "death by hysteria" after the United States entered World War I, when it was linked to pro-German sentiment or subversive radicalism by physicians opposed to it (Burrow, 1977; Numbers, 1978).

The absence of communication between medicine and social science in the 1920s was reflected in articles in both medical and economics journals. The broadening of the definition of medical economics to include the theories and methods of professional economists ceased abruptly. Although the number of articles published each year in medical journals on economic subjects remained about the same as before the war, the proportion devoted to medical income and business practices in existing journals increased sharply. The magazine *Medical Economics,* which began to publish in 1923, was unambiguously about physicians as businessmen and purchasers of expensive consumer goods. Several subjects that had begun to attract physicians' attention in the first decade of the century were excluded entirely from medical journals in the 1920s: for instance, the relation between services and the standard of living, insurance, and the role of medical care in industry.

Economists also turned their attention elsewhere. The *Index of Economic Articles* lists no papers during the 1920s on medical care or health insurance in the professional journals published by economists in the United States. Notable exceptions were the studies of the costs of illness to individuals and society, conducted by statisticians employed in the life insurance industry (Dublin and Lotka, 1930).

The separation of medicine and economics, however, cannot be ascribed entirely to physicians. Economists were not as rigorously analytical about the relation of research to policy in health care as they were about other areas in which they worked. The economists' contributions to discussions of health affairs, and their publications dealing with railroad rates, tariffs, wages, and the costs of agriculture, industry, and trade, show a striking difference in rigor. When Henry Farnam discussed the economic consequences of alcoholism or Irving Fisher the causes of national vitality, for instance, they used economists' analytical skills but justified their com-

mitments on matters of public policy on grounds other than those
they derived from analysis. Farnam, advising the Committee of Fifty
on the control of alcoholism in 1903, asserted that "economic
forces" could become "effective allies of the moral agencies which
are attacking the evils of the liquor habit" (Billings et al., 1905: 34).
Similarly, Fisher, in the concluding chapter of *A Report on National
Vitality,* quoted Ralph Waldo Emerson's statement that "Health is
the first wealth" for authority and relegated to a footnote the names
of fifteen economists who over a period of three centuries had
"included health in the category of wealth" (Fisher, 1909: 124). In
his major economic treatise, moreover, Fisher disparaged the
arguments about the value of human beings he made in his polemical
works as "of more theoretical than practical moment" (Fisher, 1906;
1930: 17).

This separation of professional and public roles can be explained only in part by the absence of a tradition of economic
analysis of health services. Many economists' concern with health
was deeply personal. Fisher, for example, believed that his father's
long illness and his own experience with tuberculosis gave him
special insight into how to improve vigor. Most of the scholars who
advocated compulsory insurance were passionately opposed to the
harsh labor practices in many American industries. The separation
between professional and polemic roles, however, was more than
personal; it also reflected the increasingly dominant professional
goal of objectivity in research. After World War I, as new
developments in economic theory and methodology reinforced the
striving for objectivity, economic research for a time became distinct
from inquiry in the broad fields of public health and medical care,
which looked toward reform.

American public health physicians, who were also aware of
European models and familiar with economists' writing on insurance, immigration, and municipal reform, were not particularly
impressed by economic analysis applied to health issues. In the late
nineteenth century, many public health physicians accepted the
premise that, as Edward Jarvis of Massachusetts wrote in 1874, the
State should assure the "power of the people to create value and
capital" (Jarvis, 1874: 373). By the second decade of the twentieth
century, some public health physicians were uneasy about such
reliance on economics. To Charles Chapin, the influential superin-
tendent of health of Providence, R.I., for example, economists were

naive about how society worked and what physicians could achieve. In 1912, Chapin challenged the practical value of the argument that the costs of preventive medical care and industrial safety would be repaid to society because workers would live longer and be more productive. Workers were not regarded as highly by industry as they were by economists. As a result of a deliberate policy of unrestricted immigration, there were more workers than jobs. This surplus of labor combined with exploitative conditions of work to produce in most citizens "an instinctive feeling that . . . a human being is not a very valuable machine." Moreover, philanthropy rather than tax revenue was a partial substitute for lost wages to families suffering untimely illness and death. Finally, Chapin warned against overconfidence in the power of medical science. Increased public investment in prevention might not produce results because the effectiveness of most preventive measures was "by no means certain" (Chapin, 1913: 104).

The Estrangement of Economists from Health Affairs, 1920–1940

In the 1920s and 1930s, the medical and economics professions became further estranged than they had been when Chapin paid sufficient attention to economists' arguments to dispute them. One result of the bitter controversy over compulsory health insurance was the assumption made both by leading physicians and by social scientists in health affairs that economics was pertinent mainly to the single issue of financing medical services.

The economists' relative lack of interest in medical care in this period, however, was a result of the internal history of the discipline as well as of the intellectual insularity of medicine. Important contributions to economic theory distracted professional attention from applications of the discipline. Beginning in England in the late 1920s, the dominant issue in economic thought became the establishment of what has been described as the macroeconomic viewpoint. As Donald Winch observed, the "central formal problems of economics, namely scarcity, value, choice, resource allocation and efficiency," ceased for a time to be the principal concerns of many leading economists (Winch, 1969; 18, 323–324). Only in retrospect does theoretical work on microeconomic problems during this period bear on health and medical issues. The most important contributions during the interim years with later bearing on medical issues were the dethronement of perfect competition as the central generalization in the theory of value and the development of a new welfare economics. But these developments were not applied effectively to practical problems for some years.

Moreover, economists increasingly separated the advocacy of reform from research and analysis in their professional activities. Like other social scientists, although concerned with social problems, in their research they became both more specialized and increasingly neutral toward proposed reforms during the middle decades of the century. In Edward Purcell's words, the "instrument of social research came to overwhelm the goal of social reform" (Purcell, 1973: 25).

In large part because economists were the first social scientists to make use of sophisticated statistical techniques, methodology replaced moral purpose in their work more quickly than it did in other disciplines. In economics, as in other social and natural sciences, the growing sophistication in methodology both derived from and reinforced the concept of multiple causality. Many economists who entered the profession in the 1920s were uneasy about the research methods and the social reform interests of many of their teachers. Economists became relativists about ethics and public policy in their professional work, generally while retaining strong personal convictions. In contrast to sociology or political science, for example, sophisticated history can be written about modern economic thought on the assumption that "the philosophical beliefs of economists are not relevant to the validity of the economic hypotheses they advance" (Blaug, 1978: 5). However, such beliefs are relevant to the choice of questions for research and the use of ambiguous evidence when economists take positions on policy.

The research conducted for the Committee on the Costs of Medical Care (CCMC) in the early 1930s, though often called economics, had little in common with the mainstream of professional economics of the time. The staff of the CCMC collected data using methods developed by economists and statisticians in the insurance industry, at the National Bureau of Economic Research, and by social scientists in such federal agencies as the Children's Bureau, the Bureau of Labor Statistics, and the departments of

Agriculture and Commerce. Most of the analysis that appeared in the committee's publications was performed by men and women trained in other fields, or by economists acting in general rather than professional roles. I.S. Falk, for example, had taught bacteriology before joining the CCMC. Although C. Rufus Rorem and Maurice Leven had doctorates in economics, Rorem was listed as a "professor of accountancy" in the progress reports of the CCMC and Leven was identified only as a "statistician." Louis Webster Jones and Louis Reed, though economists, prepared mainly descriptive studies for the committee.

The chairman of the CCMC, Ray Lyman Wilbur, despite his experience as president of Stanford University and secretary of the interior in the Hoover administration believed, like most physicians, that economics was entirely a practical tool to improve the financing of medical services. Explaining the work of the committee to medical audiences, Wilbur claimed that his purpose was to devise "a financial system by which all members of society, regardless of economic status, may receive a full or even a reasonable share of the benefits possible through modern scientific medicine." Wilbur wanted research to provide the "evidence" to develop a "modern plan" to finance the cost of medical services (Wilbur, 1928: 1–2). Economics provided useful methods to gather this evidence for medicine, in the same way that "a modern business has its statisticians and its economists surveying the past and the present and preparing for the future" (Wilbur, 1929: 1411).

Both the goals of the CCMC and the commitments of its research staff inhibited critical questions about several important assumptions. The committee staff, like Wilbur, assumed that financing and organization were the central unresolved issues in health affairs. Most of them believed that medical care needed to be reorganized to replace individual with group practice and fee-for-service with prepayment in order to permit financing through insurance. These assumptions obscured a more basic belief: that more accessible medical care would lead to improved health and social progress. Economists could not accept these assumptions as legitimate bases for research.

Since the eighteenth century, most leading economists have asserted that the intrinsic worth of what is produced, distributed, and consumed is irrelevant for economic analysis. Beginning with classic arguments by Mandeville and Bentham about the independence of morality and economic logic, members of the profession have generally ignored the social value of what is traded in any market. This aspect of economists' stance was reinforced after about 1870 when "economics . . . became largely a study of the principles that govern the efficient allocation of resources when both resources and wants are given" (Blaug, 1978: 4). With the exception of work by a small number of "institutional" economists, mainly at Columbia and the University of Wisconsin, the systematic assessment of the worth of allocations in the public sector by economists emerged, as cost-benefit analysis, only after World War II.

The authors of the studies published by the CCMC were anything but neutral about the social value of medical care. For most of them, medical science and technology were progressive and had a benevolent influence on society. This assumption permitted them to argue that reforms that made more medical care available to more people, with costs shared more equitably between individuals and society, were in the public interest.

The effects of these assumptions on the use of economics in research sponsored by the CCMC are worth examining as a case study in the application of the social sciences to health affairs. The history of the committee's recommendations for reform, and of the role of the staff and committee members in working on their behalf, is a different and important subject. There is no necessary connection between research and reform, particularly in the period since the 1920s.

The authors of research reports for the CCMC were explicit about their assumptions. Early in their study of *The Crisis in Hospital Finance,* for example, Michael Davis, a member of the committee who had trained in sociology and psychology at Columbia University, and Rorem asserted that changes in the "economic relations" between physicians and the public "are due mostly to the very advances in medicine which have so increased its power and its potentialities" (Davis and Rorem, 1932: 45). Changes in society, they asserted, were subordinate to changes in medical science as determinants of economic relations between physicians and patients. Since the eighteenth century, in contrast, most economists had regarded changes in the size and structure of the market as the principal determinants of economic relations.

Roger Irving Lee, a physician who had been deeply involved in the campaign for compulsory health insurance before World War I, and Lewis Webster Jones, a statistician and economist, emphasized medical need in their influential CCMC study, *The Fundamentals of Good Medical Care*. Their criteria for measuring how much medical care should be available were based entirely on physicians' expert opinions. The Lee-Jones study was used for a generation as the standard source of criteria of medical need in research, planning, and, in the Hill-Burton program, for public policy on the construction of hospitals.

Lee and Jones distinguished but were not particularly concerned about the difference between need and demand. A purely medical definition of the need for care was valid, they argued, only in a "society which, like our own, believes in the desirability of health and the efficacy of scientific medicine in promoting and maintaining it." Unlike India, for example, "modern America . . . has accepted . . . medicine as the proper instrument" for the "advancement" of health. In India, by contrast, a medical definition of need "would bear no relation to the 'needs' of society." Need was relative only among societies. Within each society it was absolute and best determined by medical opinion, Lee and Jones implied. It followed that there was an intricate relationship between need and demand. Although they identified the problem, they did not pursue it (Lee and Jones, 1933: 12).

In *The Cost of Medical Care,* Falk, Rorem, and Martha D. Ring were ambivalent about the relevance of economics for the analysis of health services. They introduced the economic concept of effective demand as part of their argument in favor of redistributive justice in medical care. Moreover, they considered the dilemmas created by health care as "an esoteric economic commodity concerning which the buyer has no basis for critical judgment." But they later blurred this point, declaring that because health care is a "personal service" it is not entirely an "economic commodity" (Falk, Rorem, and Ring, 1933: ix, 384, 386).

This ambivalence needs further analysis. It may have been the result of inadequate understanding of economic theory. More likely it was the result of a clash of viewpoints among the collaborators. Their differing assumptions about economics and health care were explicit in later works. Falk had a profound belief in the potential contributions of medicine and science to human welfare. These contributions, he declared in 1936, meant that "life has been given a certainty and a safety and health and human vigor have been given a reality such as were undreamed of before" (Falk, 1936: 4–5). This point of view made it difficult for Falk to be patient with economic analysis that assumed that relations between producers and consumers could be described without regard to the intrinsic value of what was exchanged.

Rorem, in contrast, perceived that the philosophical basis of economics provided insight into human behavior in health affairs just as it did in other transactions. In 1939, for example, he described and endorsed the pessimistic view of human nature on which economists' logic has been based since the eighteenth century. "Economists have known for some time," he asserted, that "emotion frequently transcends reason in the normal life and decisions of the so-called economic man" (Rorem, 1939: 84).

Louis Reed appears to have been the only staff member who doubted the strongly held beliefs of his colleagues in a CCMC publication. Concluding his monograph on *The Ability to Pay for Medical Care,* Reed (1933) expressed reservations about the context in which his data would be analyzed. "Adequate medical care and a minimum standard of living," he argued, "are . . . crude and inexact tools with which to work." The content of both concepts "depends upon and varies with the prevailing level of culture" (pp. 95–96). Moreover, ability to pay for medical care is "unsubstantial and intangible." This tentativeness stands in sharp contrast with most other general statements in the CCMC publications. To take just one, Falk asserted in *The Incidence of Illness and the Receipt and Costs of Medical Care Among Representative Families* that "the people need substantially larger volumes of medical service than they now receive; this applies equally, if not with equal force, to the well-to-do and the rich as to the poor and the very poor" (Falk, Klem, and Sinai, 1933: 247). Walton Hamilton, an academic economist who served as a member of the CCMC, exemplified the difference between the committee's staff and the economics profession in his personal statement at the end of the committee's final report. "A sharp distinction between the technology of medicine and its organization is essential to adequate analysis," he asserted. "The failure of the [Final] Report to make that distinction . . . obscures the lines of the argument" *(Medical Care for the American People,* 1932: 190). Hamilton, like Reed, believed that economists must separate the standards that governed research from those that determined their prescriptions for society.

Most of the writers on health affairs in the 1930s who had some familiarity with economics were not enthusiastic about economists' assumptions. Economists were regarded ambivalently as sources of both insight and error. Hugh Cabot, for instance, surgeon, medical school dean, and author of an influential book in 1935, *The Doctor's Bill,* both caricatured and embraced economics. Cabot, who despite his eminence was vilified within the medical profession for supporting compulsory health insurance, accused a typical economist of being, like "economic man," a "cold, detached person, apt to overlook the fact that the people affected by his plans are liable to be human beings." But Cabot also applied economic concepts, setting aside questions of the worth of medical services, to such problems as the adequacy of the supply of physicians and differential fees (Cabot, 1935: viii, 250).

An ironic result of the research and recommendations of the Committee on the Costs of Medical Care was the creation in the period 1931–1932 by the American Medical Association of the Bureau of Medical Economics. The bureau was the mirror image of the committee. Its staff, like the committee's, believed in the "overriding social importance of the nation's progress in conquering disease." The bureau, like the committee, produced thorough, quantitative reports. Bureau staff apparently cooperated with Falk and Edgar Sydenstricker, formerly on the CCMC staff, to prepare background papers for the Committee on Economic Security, appointed by President Franklin D. Roosevelt in 1934 to draft what became the Social Security Act. But the bureau staff believed that their research supported the views of organized medicine about the financing and organization of medical care. Even under the direction of a former professor of economics, Frank G. Dickinson, after 1946, the bureau issued forceful polemics as well as accurate reports. Like the CCMC staff, the bureau staff and most other medical care and public health researchers of the generation could not conceive of research that was independent of advocacy (Burrow, 1963: 184, 192, 202, 355, 360).

The only economic treatise in the 1930s to examine medicine without concern for the intrinsic value of health services was unpublished for nearly a decade. In 1937, Milton Friedman, working at first under the direction of and later as senior collaborator with Simon Kuznets at the National Bureau of Economic Research, took charge of a study of income from independent professional practice.

Friedman and Kuznets (1945) argued that physicians had a greater return on their services than other professionals, a difference that was explained only by the deliberate restriction of entry into the profession. The study was submitted as Friedman's doctoral dissertation, but it was not published until 1945. It is not clear why publication was delayed. Leonard Silk, paraphrasing Friedman, believes that the manuscript, despite elaborate statistical analysis, worried "some members of the Bureau [who] regarded this as an attack on the American medical profession" (Silk, 1976: 61). Another view is that publication was delayed first by a painfully slow review process, which required the board of directors of the bureau to approve all manuscripts for accuracy and technical merit, and then by the distractions of the war (Klarman, 1979).

Friedman and Kuznets regarded the effectiveness of physicians' services and the justice of their distribution as separate from economic analysis. Had the manuscript been published in the 1930s it would have dismayed both partisans of the CCMC report and their bitter opponents in the medical profession. The study, unique for its time, foreshadowed later developments: it became, in Herbert Klarman's (1979) words, the "dominant intellectual stream in academic economics about health." Nevertheless, the study contains the basis of Friedman's later advocacy of the abolition of state licensure of physicians in order to challenge the monopoly of organized medicine.

Economists' Involvement in Health Affairs, 1945–1960

Since World War II, most economists studying medical care and physicians' behavior have rejected a normative definition of the "economic problem" as the "wider distribution of medical care to the general population," as Sydenstricker (1935: 574) phrased it, in favor of a focus on alternative ways to allocate scarce resources to competing claimants. The Friedman-Kuznets study foreshadowed this change. By the time it appeared, however, a few economists were studying health and medical affairs as the source of unusual problems in welfare theory and microeconomics.

This change, like most historical themes, is clearer in retrospect than it was to contemporaries. Most of the medical profession, for example, even those involved in education and public health, continued to ignore economists. A paper on "Who Should Teach Health Economics?" and a lengthy discussion following it, given at a conference at the University of Michigan in 1946, did not even examine the possibility that economists should be involved, consulted, or even read (Proceedings, 1947).

Two panel discussions on the "Economics of Medical Care" at the 1950 meeting of the American Economic Association (AEA) signalled increased interest in the subject in the economics profession. According to Klarman (1979), the panels were organized by Friedman, at the request of Frank Knight, his colleague at the University of Chicago and president-elect that year of the AEA. Introducing the sessions, Eli Ginzberg understated the importance of the occasion for the study of health services by economists. He noted that for the "first time in the past two decades" the AEA was sponsoring sessions on medical care. The 1950 sessions, however, were the first in the history of the AEA since its founding in 1887 (Ginzberg, 1951).

The papers and discussions at the 1950 AEA sessions exemplify the tension between analysis of resource allocation and advocacy of reform as the focus of economists' work in health. Ginzberg argued that, although professional economists' interest in health services was stimulated by public concern with the cost of care, changes in the financing of personal health services would have little effect on the health of individuals. He told the AEA, as he had argued more forcefully in a study of hospital facilities in New York State a year earlier, that the "striking advances" of biomedical science created false optimism about the role of medical care in improving the well-being of individuals (Ginzberg, 1949). During World War II, he asserted, improvements in the standard of living of low-income groups led to improved health, despite the withdrawal of forty percent of the physicians from civilian practice. For Ginzberg, the study of health and medical issues was a problem in both economic analysis and the strategy of reform in social policy.

Several participants in the AEA sessions preferred analysis to advocacy. Klarman, writing on "Requirements for Physicians," challenged the assumptions about estimating needs for medical services in the Lee-Jones study for the CCMC. He advocated a standard of requirements for physicians that took into account "economic costs in the sense of alternatives foregone." Requirements for care were not exclusively determined by what medical science could deliver if only the barriers of finance and organization were removed (Klarman, 1951: 644). Jerome Rothenberg (1951) of Amherst College applied welfare economics to the problems of financing medical care; his paper, with hindsight, foreshadows Kenneth Arrow's (1963) paper on medical care and the economics of uncertainty. C.A. Kulp (1951) of the Wharton School analyzed the potential effects of different combinations of compulsory and of voluntary health insurance.

Unlike Kulp, Klarman, and Rothenberg, the participants in the second AEA panel, "Alternative Solutions," assumed that the means to provide more and better health services were known, rather than that alternative ways to allocate resources needed further analysis. Seymour Harris of Harvard defended the achievements of the British National Health Services against its American critics (Harris, 1951). Frank Dickinson, of the American Medical Association Bureau of Economic Research, asserted that the existing organization and financing of medical services in the United States were appropriate because the productivity of physicians was increasing and their fees were rising more slowly than the rate of inflation (Dickinson, 1951).

The most prominent controversies about health issues in the economics literature of the late 1940s and 1950s involved advocacy of public policy rather than analysis of alternative interpretations of the behavior of the health industry and the allocation of resources to and within it. For instance, Ginzberg and Harris disagreed in the *American Economic Review* about the value of the recommendations of the 1952 report by the President's Commission on the Health Needs of the Nation (Ginzberg, 1954; Harris, 1954). Falk debated with Glen and Rita Campbell about the merits of compulsory health insurance, in the *Quarterly Journal of Economics*. The tension between advocacy and analysis as the primary goals of scholars who applied economic thought and methods to health services, first evident in the late 1930s, persisted two decades later.

Events in economics and in the health sector in the 1940s and 1950s seem, with hindsight, to account for the rapid expansion of interest among economists in research on the behavior of the health industry in the 1960s. It is plausible, though it cannot be demonstrated, that the size of the industry and the ferment within it attracted economists' attention. The health sector of the general economy expanded vigorously in the 1950s. Expenditures for new facilities and for hospital services increased sharply. Physicians' incomes began to rise faster than those of other professionals. Moreover, information collected by public and private agencies in order to plan, regulate, and justify new programs created data resources that could be used for economic analysis.

Events particular to economics as a discipline contributed to the interest in health affairs. These events included the growing prestige of the economics profession, the application of economic analysis to problems of defense and foreign affairs, a growing professional interest in public finance as a field in which to apply new theories and methods in welfare economics, microeconomics and econometrics, and the interest of labor economists in medical care as a fringe benefit and in the health of the labor force. Although it is not clear how much importance should be attached to each of these events, they are evident in much of the economics literature on health services and medical care published in the 1960s.

The prestige of economists in public affairs increased in the 1940s and 1950s. Their theories and methods of research contributed in useful ways to such matters as mitigating business cycles, predicting and understanding changes in production and consumption, assisting in negotiations between management and labor, and clarifying problems of military strategy and tactics (Norton, 1969). By the 1970s, the distinction between macro- and microeconomics came to apply mainly to the problems economists engaged in rather than to a difference between the public and the private sectors.

The discipline of economics appeared to be expansive, affluent, and self-assured. Most economists who entered the profession after the 1950s have had little reason to inquire into the history of their discipline or to notice, for example, that the influence of economists on public policy has varied widely in different nations at different times over the past several centuries. Economists have developed enormous confidence in the power of the theory and methods developed since the 1920s to clarify choices among competing public policies. As Martin Feldstein (1967: 1), to take but one example, wrote in 1967, with more assurance than historical accuracy, only after World War II had economists developed "optimizing methods that indicate appropriate policies subject to behavioral and technical constraints." By limiting his historical view to formal mathematical methods of optimizing, Feldstein passed over considerable economic analysis applied to public policy.

The areas of public policy in which economists' involvement after 1945 had the fewest historical precedents were defense, health, and education (Fein, 1971; Dunlop, 1979). There are striking similarities between the economics of war and of health and education. In these fields, large public investment, in a period when the prestige of the discipline was high, created opportunities for economists to deal with issues that had previously been regarded as in the domain of other professions. In defense, health, and education, moreover, economists' involvement in public affairs began before the new subject matter achieved academic legitimacy. Economists in defense, health, and education agencies, employed mainly as staff generalists rather than as economists, wrote memoranda and reports for committees and public officials before they wrote papers on these subjects for their professional journals.

Mobilization for war made it respectable for scholars to write bureaucratic papers without being stigmatized by their peers for not producing scholarly work. Similarly, increased public investment in health care and frequent assertions of crisis since the 1960s helped to make an interest in health affairs acceptable among academic economists. The health care crisis was, in a way, the professional equivalent of the Cold War.

The issues faced by economists in health and in defense are similar. In both fields, economists become absorbed in a single industry in which life or death results from an output of services, and numerous situations occur in which the market paradigm operates imperfectly or not at all. Both fields require expertise in the analysis of externalities, of productivity, and of substitution. In the 1960s, these similarities became more than analogies useful for comprehending intellectual history, when a few economists began to work in both health and defense studies (Hitch and McKean, 1967; Smith, 1966; Schlesinger, 1963).

The analogy between the health care crisis of the 1960s and 1970s and war as stimuli for economic research should not be exaggerated. During the 1950s, economic research on health affairs was stimulated by earlier work by Friedman and Kuznets on professional income, encouraged by Seymour Harris's interest in public policy for financing services, and was beginning to emerge in the work of John Dunlop and his students at Harvard. Other economists whose contributions to the field began before health became a major focus of public attention and investment in the 1960s included Robert Lampman, Tibor Scitovsky, and Burton Weisbrod. Selma Mushkin (1958) summarized some of these trends in research. In 1960, while a staff member of the Ford Foundation, Victor Fuchs commissioned the manuscripts that were published as Kenneth Arrow's (1963) paper, "Uncertainty and the Welfare Economics of Medical Care," and an overview of the field by Klarman (1965), *Economics of Health*.

The growth of interest in health affairs among economists was more strongly influenced by the study of public finance and by labor economics than by the study of military and defense issues. Students of public finance and labor, moreover, have long been aware of the tension between advocacy and analysis as purposes for economics. For the first four decades of this century, research both in labor economics and in the promotion of public policy to regulate collective bargaining and provide social insurance was identified with John R. Commons and his students at the University of Wisconsin. Two of Commons's colleagues who worked in public finance, Edwin F. Witte and Arthur Altmeyer, became central figures in the creation of the Social Security program in the 1930s and 1940s. Their relations with the medical care researchers from the CCMC research staff who joined the Social Security Board (later Administration)— Agnes Brewster, Falk, Margaret Klem, and Reed—were important to the development of interest in health economics and of government support for health services research using the methods of economics. The Wisconsin tradition in the study of public finance was reflected in the work of Klarman, Lampman, and Weisbrod, and was an important influence on such papers as "A Formula for Social Insurance Financing," by Selma Mushkin and Anne Scitovsky (1945) in the *American Economic Review*.

The growing importance of health care as a fringe benefit during and after World War II attracted the attention of economists as researchers and advisers to industry, unions, and government. Dunlop of Harvard, the most influential labor economist of his generation, was, through Sumner Slichter, an heir to aspects of the Wisconsin tradition. He recalled that "[my] interest in . . . medical care began when I found myself . . . in a position of having to propose whether to spend $250,000,000 of the railroad's money on health and welfare programs" (Dunlop, 1965: 1325). The problem Dunlop encountered as, in his phrase, a "neutral participant" in labor management disputes—how much money, spent for what ser-

vices, would produce what results—became a subject for research by
other labor economists, and served as the basis for the creation of a
loosely organized group of scholars at Harvard and elsewhere who
worked on problems in the economics of health. As Joseph Garbarino, a student of Dunlop's who was teaching at Berkeley, wrote in
1960, to ignore the question of how medical care could be more
effectively organized and financed meant using the "union's bargaining position to win benefits for the medical profession and the
hospitals" (Garbarino, 1960: 35).

A number of economists concluded that medical fees and
hospital income were rising in the 1950s as a result of the "pressure
of a growing demand for medical care on an inelastic supply of services" (Garbarino, 1959). By the early 1960s, the optimistic proposition urged by economists employed by the American Medical
Association, that medical productivity was increasing faster than
fees, had been refuted by both labor economists and scholars,
notably Reuben Kessel (1958), who extended the Friedman-Kuznets
analysis to the problem of price discrimination by monopolies.

Other economists elaborated the contemporary variant of the
theory of human capital. Mushkin, a leading promoter as well as an
astute recent historian of the study of human capital, described the
"primary question" in this field as "the contribution of changes in
the quality of people to economic growth" (Mushkin, 1962: 93).
More than any other area of economics involving health affairs, the
study of human capital is linked to a long history of work in adjacent
disciplines, notably statistics and epidemiology. Moreover, the implications of data on the amount, variety, distribution, and cost of
illness for sanitation, preventive medicine, and social policy toward
the poor have been matters of debate for several centuries.

The proposition that improvements in the standard of living and
the availability of services increase the economic value of the average
person was an attractive bridge between analysis and advocacy of
reform in the 1950s and 1960s. This proposition, articulated by
William Petty in the seventeenth century, had appealed to
Benthamite reformers in early nineteenth-century England and to
the economists who supported compulsory health insurance in the
United States before World War I. For Mushkin and other
economists employed by the federal government or by state and
voluntary health agencies in the 1950s and early 1960s, the theory of
human capital justified collaboration both with professional

economists and with medical care reformers who, like Falk and Davis, continued to press for compulsory health insurance, what Daniel Hirshfield (1970) called the "lost reform" of the 1930s.

The compatibility of concern about human capital and dedication to improved access to personal health services was demonstrated in numerous studies published by the Social Security Administration or presented at the annual meetings of the Medical Care Section of the American Public Health Association during the 1950s and early 1960s. Mushkin, surveying this work after the first national conference on health economics in 1962, was delighted with the growing interest in the "ways in which the improved health of the people contributes to enlarging the resources and output of an economy" (*The Economics of Health and Medical Care,* 1964: 3).

Studies of human capital made the application of economic analysis to health issues less controversial because they subsumed the controversial issue of how to finance medical care under the larger question of the benefits of improved health. In the first two decades of the century, Fisher, collaborating with statisticians, had taken advantage of a similar strategic opportunity to promote both research and compulsory health insurance. In the 1950s and early 1960s, economic writing in this tradition provided some of the intellectual justification for legislation to expand access to health services for the elderly and the poor, as well as a source of research problems that were widely respected among academic economists.

Rashi Fein, in a 1958 monograph for the Commission on Mental Illness, *The Economics of Mental Illness,* demonstrated both the application of the study of human capital to social policy and the ambiguity of the relation between research and advocacy of reform. For Fein, morality was both independent of and, in some circumstances, a deduction from economic logic. Moral principles had a major role in guiding the "institutions that society has established for the ultimate purpose of caring for and advancing the members of that society." But moral ends could be achieved by economic means under certain conditions. Introducing the concept of relative abundance, a notion explored by a handful of economists over the past several centuries, Fein conjectured a "world in which the using of resources in a particular way does not come . . . at the expense of other uses, but instead increases the total supply of resources available." In such a world, Fein argued, a moral act, such as increasing expenditures for the care of the mentally ill, could also be an efficient act because it would "reduce the indirect costs by more than the direct expenditures were increased" (Fein, 1958: 127, 129–130).

Unlike Mushkin and Fein, however, economists, particularly in the twentieth century, have seldom considered changes over time in the human condition to be pertinent to theory and its applications. Economics has been viewed from within the discipline mainly as the rigorous study of the allocation of scarce resources among competing wants. Moral considerations have usually been regarded as relevant only when economists decided that the market had ceased to operate properly. When the market appeared to operate properly, economic principles, most economists have assumed, were the best rules a society could follow. Before the twentieth century, however, as Dunlop notes, it was "not possible so sharply to separate the policy prescriptions of economists which typically in part include normative elements and the technical and formal analysis of the discipline" (Dunlop, 1979).

Economists and Health Affairs Since 1960

When historians of economic thought study the recent application of economics to health affairs, they may regard the early 1960s as a period of ferment after which the traditional concerns of economists became increasingly dominant. Arrow's 1963 paper, "Uncertainty and the Welfare Economics of Medical Care," may be viewed as a symbolic event. Arrow connected the economics of health to mathematical economic analysis and the most sophisticated welfare economics. He advocated the paradigm of the market, modified by uncertainty that justified unusual intervention, as the basis for studying the differences between health and other industries.

The ascendancy of conventional economic analysis in health affairs can also be measured by the differences in the contributions to two national conferences on health economics, in 1962 and 1968. At the first conference, concerns about human capital and economic development framed the papers and discussions. The papers, which were presented by economists and people who worked more broadly in public health, discussed practical issues in organizing and financing care, the cost and efficiency of hospitals, and the evaluation of programs. The papers used mainly qualitative methods. In 1968, Klarman, who edited the papers presented at the second conference, noted that the contributors worked with the dominant, mainly mathematical methods and concepts of the discipline. Only economists were invited to present papers. Moreover, the planning committee decided to ignore the "recent increase in health services costs . . . and the sources and mechanisms of financing health services" (Klarman, 1970: 12). Although some of the participants in the 1962 conference were present in 1968, none presented papers and several were critical of the complex methodology and the lack of relevance to public issues of the work presented.

Between 1962 and 1968 a larger number of professional economists, supported by increasing public and foundation funds, worked on problems of the health sector than ever before. A substantial amount of completed research and orderly data was available by the late 1950s, in large part as a result of work within the Social Security Administration and grants from other agencies in the federal government. In the early 1960s, research on economics was funded by the National Institutes of Health (NIH) and the Division of Community Health Services (DCHS) of the Bureau of State Services in the Public Health Service. Agnes Brewster, chief of the Health Economics Branch of the DCHS, had served with the CCMC staff and the research group in the Social Security Administration. Other research in health economics was funded by the Division of Hospitals and Medical Facilities in the Hill-Burton program. In 1968, these activities were consolidated in the new National Center for Health Services Research and Development (Sloat, 1978).

In 1965, Herman and Anne Somers, in a paper prepared for the Brookings Institution and the Public Health Service, argued that "professional economists, by and large, have not played a major role in the study of health care issues." By 1967, when their paper was published, this pessimism was no longer justified.

In that year, to take a significant example, the Committee on Chronic Kidney Disease created by the Bureau of the Budget adopted as a recommendation for policy the results of a paper by Klarman and Gerald Rosenthal, both members of the committee, applying cost-effectiveness analysis to competing methods of treatment for end-stage renal disease (Gottshalk, 1967). Moreover, the Gottshalk Committee and later the Congress accepted their recommendation that dialysis be financed by a variety of programs, with "major reliance" for operating costs on Title XVIII of the Social Security Act.

After about 1968, health economics was securely established within both the discipline of economics and the broader field of health research. Since that time, the history of economic analysis of health affairs has been less a study of landmarks than a record of increased interest in the subject among economists, of growing public investment in research and training, of the rapid growth of a scholarly literature, and of vigorous disputes about theory, methods, and applications similar to those in other areas of economists' concern. Moreover, largely as a result of increased economic research, economists have been consulted with growing frequency by officials of government and private agencies concerned with health policy. The tension between advocacy and analysis persists, although the balance of effort and investment has shifted to the latter.

Health economics benefited to some extent from events that affected social science in general. Government support for social science research increased in the 1960s as the result of a widely held assumption that research would make social policy more effective. The demand for faculty by new and expanding universities attracted an unprecedented number of people to graduate education. Professional economists and other social scientists in influential administrative and advisory positions in government advocated support for research and training and increased investment in testing the feasibility of new programs and evaluating existing ones. Discontent with United States involvement in Vietnam may have attracted some scholars, particularly graduate students, from defense to health studies, or at least to alternative service in the Public Health Service.

Health economics was less important than either the legacy of reform or electoral politics in framing the major health legislation of the 1960s. Klarman recalled in 1977 that "we all missed the effects of Medicare and Medicaid—wrong on use and on cost or price." This judgment may be too harsh. Medicare was a political victory for the medical care reform coalition originally organized in the 1930s. The victory was made possible by the Democratic landslide of 1964. After members of this group decided to move incrementally toward national health insurance, little new research, in contrast to the amount of political organizing activity, was required (Marmor, 1973).

Klarman (1970: 9), describing the participants in the 1968 conference, observed that "economists who work on health service problems" seem to have a "higher level" of interest in public policy than "prevails in other applied areas of economics." This strong interest in public policy may not be unique to health economics. It seems characteristic of scholars who devote their careers to a single sector or industry. Agricultural economists have a long history of passionate involvement in farm policy and defense economists have engaged in bitter polemics about appropriate weapons and strategy. During the past two decades, however, economists working in the health field have increasingly adopted the attitude urged by Victor Fuchs in 1963: "The economists can suggest some of the questions that ought to be asked. They cannot give the answers. The answers have to come out of the health field itself" (Conference on Research in Hospital Use, 1963: 74).

Health economists' concern for public policy should be considered in the context of the development of broad political unity among social scientists in the past generation. Social scientists in general have become more concerned with research than with advocacy of reform since the 1920s. This shift was reflected in the dominance of pluralist ideology in the 1950s and 1960s. This viewpoint was exemplified by Odin Anderson, writing in 1966 on the "Influence of Social and Economic Research on Public Policy in the Health Field." Anderson advocated both a normative basis for applied research and a scholarly neutrality toward the organization of the health sector. On the one hand, he argued that useful applied research required a "consensus" among scholars, which provided a "framework for research bearing on policy." He found this consensus in the concept of the desirability of equal access to health services. On the other hand, writing autobiographically, Anderson claimed that he and his colleagues adopted a "strategy" of "accepting the prevailing health services and health insurance structure as given," and then examining "deviations from or innovations in the system." A consensus could be so broad, he implied, that social scientists could proceed as if what ought to be and what is were synonymous (Anderson, 1966: 11, 31, 39).

The pluralist view of American society, admittedly oversimplified here, assumes a broad social consensus about the goals of individuals and of groups. Various groups are viewed as contending according to generally accepted rules for a share of the nation's growing resources. Social imperfections yield, in time, to the pressures of intergroup competition. As critics on the Left have noted in recent years, pluralism encourages toleration of social imperfections as temporary. Injustice and inequality are regarded as normal; they can be ameliorated by group pressure over time. In Edward Purcell's (1973: 271–272) words, pluralism has provided a "logical passageway" that enables many scholars to accept "an ideology that in fact served to justify a quite imperfect *status quo*." Some critics believe that socialization within academic disciplines, by providing rewards to those who accept the pluralist vision, transforms graduate students from potential critics to faculty members who defend existing conditions. As Robert Lekachman (1976: 183) notes, criticizing higher education in economics, "It is not cynicism which turns social science critics and intellectuals into useful technicians, it is the human process which over time assimilates self-interest to larger social purposes."

The more strongly economists working in health affairs desire close connections with their disciplinary colleagues, the more likely they are to adopt pluralist views about alternative policies to finance and organize health and medical services. Unlike the researcher-reformers in medical care in the 1930s, who were detached from academic disciplines, the health economists of the 1960s and 1970s have increasingly conducted their careers in conventional academic settings, or in research organizations employing a staff of economists. In both settings, they are under strong pressures to be responsive to professional peers. The problems economists have selected for research have increasingly been derived from within the discipline or from priorities for research and policy set by regulators or observers of the health industry at the national level. Neutrality toward the claims of competing interest groups is instilled in them by their training and their relations with their peers. This neutrality, though it reinforces pluralist ideology, is generally viewed as non-ideological from within the discipline. Most professional economists agree with Mark Blaug that the study of "ruling scientific ideas" can be separated from the ideology in which they are inevitably embedded. Moreover, many scholars retain a strong conviction that neutrality about the merits of different policies is a practical fact, and that pluralism is the only useful set of assumptions about American society. As Dunlop (1979) says, "There are many competitive ideas as to 'reform.' Economic analysis may outline some of these alternative approaches . . . without advocacy of any one."

Pluralism became controversial in every social science during the 1960s. Sociologists, political scientists, psychologists, and historians, for example, debated, often bitterly, the appropriate stance of their discipline toward American institutions and public policy. Although the long-term effects on research of the debate over pluralism remain unclear, in the short run among social scientists the conflict seems to have reinforced neutrality about solutions to social problems. In the 1950s and early 1960s, relativist views about the merits of competing groups and policies were mainly ideological. Contemporary relativism, in contrast, seems also to value neutrality on controversial issues because it reduces conflicts among scholars that interfere with the enterprise of research and teaching.

Whatever the influence of pluralism in limiting advocacy of social reform among scholars, it has contributed to what may be the beginning of a striking change in the relation between medicine and the social sciences in universities. The barriers between medicine and social science that have existed in the modern university since the nineteenth century have begun to be lowered. In recent years, a few social scientists and physicians are for the first time teaching each other's students and more of them are engaging in collaborative research. The separateness of academic physicians and social scientists, rooted in philosophical and practical issues a century old, was increased in the second and third decades of this century by the bitter controversy over compulsory insurance. Physicians' mistrust of economics, when it was defined as anything except the financial management of practice, persisted through the debates about health policy from the 1930s to the 1960s. Only in the 1960s did a small number of influential physicians and social scientists begin to discover their common interest. The development of research and training in the economics of health services at Harvard is perhaps the most celebrated example of this collaboration, but similar developments occurred at other major universities. These relations might have been impossible without widespread neutrality among physicians and economists in their attitude toward competing views of how health care ought to be delivered, and in their acceptance of plural arrangements for financing and organizing care.

Analysis and the advocacy of public policy became competing goals for social scientists during this century. The tension between analysis and advocacy in disciplinary research was perpetuated rather than resolved by the creation of a field of medical care or health services research. A similar process seems to have occurred in the activities called operations research and policy analysis.

However, the choices each scholar makes about the relation between analysis and advocacy, in his or her work, are influenced by personal values and by professional and philosophical commitments. Disagreements among scholars cannot be predicted by a formula or reduced to simple categories.

In part as a legacy of recent intellectual history, most economists, like other social scientists, are relativists about solutions to social problems. Most are intensely skeptical of any proposals for reform. This skepticism often irritates people outside academic disciplines who are committed to stimulating or preventing particular changes in public policy. However, relativism has made it easier for social scientists, and for economists in particular, to collaborate with physicians, health administrators, and public officials with whom they share an ideological commitment that ideology is dangerous. This collaboration has stimulated vigorous research and teaching in recent years. However, the integration of economics and medicine in our time has had, as yet, an indeterminate effect on public policy for health care.

Note on Methods and Sources

This paper is an essay in contemporary intellectual history. Intellectual historians interested in the natural and social sciences study what Thomas Kuhn calls the "interstices between the history of science and . . . the concerns of the cultural and socioeconomic historian" (Gilbert and Graubard, 1972: 179). The subject matter of intellectual history is "states of mind" (Higham, 1961: 220). According to Felix Gilbert, "The intellectual historian reconstitutes the mind of an individual or of groups at the times when a particular event happened (Gilbert and Graubard, 1972: 155). From the late nineteenth to the mid-twentieth centuries, most historians believed that contemporary events could not be studied objectively. Many historians now explore contemporary events, but they are cautious about their conclusions. As the editors of *The Journal of Contemporary History* wrote in their first issue, "it is not the only and perhaps not the major task of the historian to pass final judgment" (Editorial Note, 1966).

Although intellectual historians often study the same sources as historians of science or of economic thought, they study them for different purposes. Like historians of science, intellectual historians are interested in the internal history of particular disciplines and in what Kuhn calls the "special role which that discipline's past always plays in its current evolution" (Gilbert and Graubard, 1972: 165, 167). But intellectual historians focus on the connections between internal history and the thought and behavior of the communities that surround workers in particular sciences. Applications of the results of scientific work, to public policy for example, are particularly useful for studying these connections.

A central analytical concept in this paper is tension. This concept is used to describe troubled or troubling relations among ideas or values. Tension is not the same as contradiction. Moreover, it is often not expressed in conflict. Rather it is a lack of coherence among ideas or values and is usually expressed as ambiguity or uneasiness. Tension can exist within disciplines, or between the theory and purposes of a discipline and ideas or values in the larger communities in which scholars work. The first use of the concept of tension analytically was by literary critics, particularly for what is generally called the "close reading" of poetry. The concept of tension was adapted to the purposes of intellectual history about forty years ago, mainly by scholars associated with the multidisciplinary field of American Studies.

In preparing this essay, I examined economists' views about the questions it was appropriate to ask and the relation between economic analysis grounded in research and advocacy of solutions to social problems. I took my definition of the work of economists from the profession itself, and from historians of economic thought. This definition permitted my research to build on existing knowledge.

Secondary sources for intellectual history and for the history of economic thought are plentiful for the years before World War II and scarce for the period since the 1940s. Particularly useful monographs describe the history of economic thought and of other social sciences in the United States and in Europe, the professionalization of the social sciences and the growth of universities, the history of medicine and of medical institutions, and the social, political, and intellectual history of political action to make health services more responsive to the conditions of industrial society.

There are several categories of primary sources. The literature of what is loosely called "medical economics" consists mainly of journals, pamphlets, books, and reports to public and voluntary organizations. This literature is classified under a variety of headings in the standard bibliographic references, beginning with the *Index Catalogue of the Library of the Surgeon General of the United States* in the nineteenth century and including *Index Medicus* and, recently, various computerized bibliographies.

Primary sources for the history of economic thought are efficiently organized. The *Index of Economic Articles* is an essential starting point for economic thought in this century. Because of the long tradition of scholarship in this field, many monographs contain useful lists of published and unpublished sources.

The most difficult primary sources to locate and interpret for the study of the application of economic thought to health services and medical care are those bearing on public policy. The large collections of public papers relating to health affairs in the United States in the past half-century have not been systematically assessed. Much of the history written about the period since the 1930s still relies on personal recollections that have not been documented. The best monographs in this area, cited in the text of the paper, are appropriately cautious.

There is considerable primary source material for the study of the developing institutional framework for research in health economics. The summaries of grants and contracts awarded by federal agencies since the early 1960s for research in economics and related fields are particularly useful. These documents, if studied in combination with the results of peer review and the administrative history of health services research, will form the basis for useful monographs in the future.

References

Allen, W. H. 1907. Hospital Efficiency. *The American Journal of Sociology* 12: 298–318.

———. 1909. *Civics and Health*. Boston, Mass.: Ginn.

American Medical Association. 1937. Suggested Outline for Course in Medical Economics. *Journal of the American Medical Association* 108: 41B–43B.

Anderson, O. W. 1966. Influence of Social and Economic Research on Public Policy in the Health Field. *Milbank Memorial Fund Quarterly/Health and Society* 44 (Summer): 11–47.

Arrow, K. J. 1963. Uncertainty and the Welfare Economics of Medical Care. *American Economic Review* 53: 941–973.

Billings, J. S., Eliot, C. W., Farnam, H. W., Greene, J. L., and Peabody, F. G. 1905. *The Liquor Problem.* Boston, Mass.: Houghton Mifflin.

Blaug, M. 1978. *Economic Theory in Retrospect.* London and New York: Cambridge University Press.

Bonner, T. N. 1963. *American Doctors and German Universities: A Chapter in International Intellectual Relations.* Lincoln, Nebr.: University of Nebraska Press.

Burns, C. R. 1977. Richard Clarke Cabot (1868–1939) and the Reformation in American Medical Ethics. *Bulletin of the History of Medicine* 51: 353–368.

Burrow, J. G. 1963. *AMA: Voice of American Medicine.* Baltimore, Md.: Johns Hopkins University Press.

————. 1977. *Organized Medicine in the Progressive Era.* Baltimore, Md.: Johns Hopkins University Press.

Cabot, H. 1935. *The Doctor's Bill.* New York: Columbia University Press.

Chapin, C. V. 1913. The Value of Human Life. *American Journal of Public Health* 3: 101–105.

Clark, G. 1971. Bernard Mandeville, M.D., and Eighteenth-Century Ethics. *Bulletin of the History of Medicine* 45: 430–443.

Conference on Research in Hospital Use. 1963. Hospital and Medical Facilities Series. Hill-Burton Program. U.S. Department of Health, Education, and Welfare. Washington, D.C.: Public Health Service.

Cowen, D. L. 1969. Liberty, Laissez-Faire and Licensure in Nineteenth-Century Britain. *Bulletin of the History of Medicine* 43: 30–40.

Cullen, M. J. 1975. *The Statistical Movement in Early Victorian Britain: The Foundations of Empirical Social Research.* New York: Harvester Press.

Dickinson, F. G. 1951. Discussion. *American Economic Review (Supplement)* 41: 688–696.

Davis, M. M., and Rorem, C. R. 1932. *The Crisis in Hospital Finance and Other Studies in Hospital Economics.* Chicago: University of Chicago Press.

Dorfman, J. 1949. *The Economic Mind in American Civilization.* Vol. 3. New York: Viking Press.

Dublin, L. I., and Lotka, A. J. 1930. *The Money Value of a Man.* New York: Ronald Press.

Dunlop, J. T. 1965. The Capacity of the United States to Provide and Finance Expanding Health Services. *Bulletin of the New York Academy of Medicine* 41: 1325–1332.

———. 1979. Letter to David P. Willis, commenting on a draft of this paper and providing these references.

The Economics of Health and Medical Care. 1964. Proceedings of the Conference on the Economics of Health and Medical Care, sponsored by the Bureau of Public Health Economics and the Department of Economics, May 10–12, 1962. University of Michigan, Ann Arbor.

Editorial Note. 1966. *Journal of Contemporary History* 1: iii-iv.

Falk, I. S. 1936. *Security Against Illnesses: A Study of Health Insurance.* Garden City, N. Y.: Doubleday Doran. Reissued 1972. New York: Da Capo Press.

———, Klem, M. C., and Sinai, N. 1933. *The Incidence of Illness and the Receipt and Costs of Medical Care among Representative Families.* Chicago: University of Chicago Press.

———, Rorem, C. R., and Ring, M. D. 1933. *The Cost of Medical Care.* Chicago: University of Chicago Press.

Fein, R. 1958. *The Economics of Mental Illness.* New York: Basic Books.

———. 1971. On Measuring Economic Benefits of Health Programs. In McLachlan, G., and McKeon, T., eds., *Medical History and Medical Care.* London: Oxford University Press.

Feldstein, M. S. 1967. *Economic Analysis for Health Service Efficiency.* Amsterdam: North Holland.

Fisher, I. N. 1906; 2nd ed., 1930. *The Nature of Capital and Income.* London and New York: Macmillan.

———. 1909. *A Report on National Vitality: Its Wastes and Conservation.* Washington, D.C.: Government Printing Office.

———. 1956. *My Father, Irving Fisher.* New York: Comet Press.

Fox, D. M. 1967. *The Discovery of Abundance: Simon N. Patten and the Transformation of Social Theory.* Ithaca, N.Y.: Cornell University Press for the American Historical Association.

———. 1979. The Segregation of Medical Ethics: A Problem in Intellectual History. *The Journal of Medicine and Philosophy* 3 (March): 81–97.

Friedman, M., and Kuznets, S. 1945. *Income from Independent Professional Practice.* New York: National Bureau of Economic Research.

Garbarino, J. W. 1959. Price Behavior and Productivity in the Medical Market. *Industrial and Labor Relations Review* 13: 4–15.

————. 1960. *Health Plans and Collective Bargaining*. Berkeley and Los Angeles: University of California Press.

Gilbert, F., and Graubard, S. R., eds. 1972. *Historical Studies Today*. New York: W.W. Norton.

Ginzberg, E. 1949. *A Pattern for Hospital Care*. New York: Columbia University Press.

————. 1951. Perspectives on the Economics of Medical Care. *American Economic Review (Supplement)* 41: 617–625.

————. 1954. What Every Economist Should Know About Health and Medicine. *American Economic Review* 44: 104–119.

Gottshalk, C. L. 1967. *Report of the Committee on Chronic Kidney Disease*. Unpublished report submitted to the director, Bureau of the Budget.

Halévy, E. 1955. *The Growth of Philosophic Radicalism*. Translated by M. Morris. Boston: Beacon Press.

Harris, S. E. 1951. The British Health Experiment. *American Economic Review (Supplement)* 41: 652–666.

————. 1954. What Every Economist Should Know About Health and Medicine: Comment. *American Economic Review* 44: 922–928.

Haskell, T. L. 1977. *The Emergence of Professional Social Science*. Urbana, Ill.: University of Illinois Press.

Herbst, J. 1965. *The German Historical School in American Scholarship*. Ithaca, N.Y.: Cornell University Press.

Higham, J. 1961. American Intellectual History: A Critical Appraisal. *American Quarterly* 13: 219–233.

Hirshfield, D. 1970. *The Lost Reform: The Campaign for Compulsory Health Insurance in the United States from 1932 to 1943*. Cambridge, Mass.: Harvard University Press.

Hitch, C. J., and McKean, R. N. 1967. *The Economics of Defense in the Nuclear Age*. Cambridge, Mass.: Harvard University Press.

Hutchinson, T. W. 1964. *'Positive' Economics and Policy Objectives*. London: Allen and Unwin.

Jarvis, E. 1874. *Political Economy of Health*. Boston, Mass.: Wright and Potter.

Kessel, R. A. 1958. Price Discrimination in Medicine. *The Journal of Law and Economics* 1: 20–53. Reprinted 1975 in Mansfield, E., ed., *Microeconomics: Selected Readings*. New York: W. W. Norton.

Klarman, H. E. 1951. Requirements for Physicians. *American Economic Review (Supplement)* 41: 633–645.

———. 1965. *The Economics of Health.* New York: Columbia University Press.

———. 1970. *Empirical Studies in Health Economics.* Baltimore: Johns Hopkins University Press.

———. 1977. Presentation on Health Economics. Unpublished paper for the Committee on Health Services Research, Institute of Medicine, National Academy of Sciences.

———. 1979. Oral commentary accompanying written comment on manuscript draft of this paper.

Kulp, C. A. 1951. Voluntary and Compulsory Medical Care Insurance. *American Economic Review (Supplement)* 41: 633–645.

Lee, R. I., and Jones, L. W. 1933. *The Fundamentals of Good Medical Care.* Chicago: University of Chicago Press.

Lekachman, R. 1976. *Economists at Bay: Why the Experts Will Never Solve Your Problems.* New York: McGraw-Hill.

Lubove, R. 1968. *The Struggle for Social Security.* Cambridge, Mass.: Harvard University Press.

Marmor, T. R. 1973. *The Politics of Medicare.* Chicago: Aldine.

McKean, R. N., ed. 1967. *Issues in Defense Economics.* New York and London: Columbia University Press for the National Bureau of Economic Research.

Medical Care for the American People: The Final Report of the Committee on the Costs of Medical Care. 1932. Chicago: University of Chicago Press.

Mini, P. V. 1974. *Philosophy and Economics: The Origins and Development of Economic Theory.* Gainesville, Fla.: University Presses of Florida.

Mushkin, S. 1958. Toward a Definition of Health Economics. *Public Health Reports* 73: 785–793.

———. 1962. Health as an Investment. *Journal of Political Economy* 70: 129–157. Reprinted in Cooper, M. H., and Culyer, A. J., eds., 1973. *Health Economics: Selected Readings.* Baltimore: Penguin Books.

———, and de Scitovzky [*sic*], A. 1945. A Formula for Social Insurance Financing. *American Economic Review* 35: 646–652.

Nelson, D. 1969. *Unemployment Insurance: The American Experience, 1915–1935.* Madison, Wis.: University of Wisconsin Press.

Norton, H. S. 1969. *The Role of Economists in Government: A Study of Economic Advice Since 1920.* Berkeley: McCutchan.

Numbers, R. 1978. *Almost Persuaded: American Physicians and Compulsory Health Insurance, 1912–1920.* Baltimore, Md.: Johns Hopkins University Press.

Proceedings of the Conference on Preventive Medicine and Health Economics, September 30–October 4, 1946. School of Public Health, University of Michigan, Ann Arbor. Mimeograph reproduction, 1947.

Purcell, E. A. 1973. *The Crisis of Democratic Theory.* Lexington, Ky.: University Press of Kentucky.

Reed, L. 1933. *The Ability to Pay for Medical Care.* Chicago: University of Chicago Press.

Roberts, D. 1960. *Victorian Origins of the British Welfare State.* New Haven, Conn.: Yale University Press.

Rorem, C. R. 1939. Mental Health and Medical Economics. *Hospitals* 13: 80–84.

Rothenberg, J. 1951. Welfare Implications of Alternative Methods of Financing Medical Care. *American Economic Review (Supplement)* 41: 676–687.

Routh, G. 1975. *The Origin of Economic Ideas.* White Plains, N.Y.: International Arts and Sciences Press.

Rubinow, I. M. 1914. The Recent Trend of Real Wages. *American Economic Review* 4: 793–817.

———. 1916. *Standards of Health Insurance.* New York: Henry Holt.

Schlesinger, J. R. Quantitative Analysis and National Security. *World Politics* 15: 295–315.

Silk, L. 1976. *The Economists.* New York: Basic Books.

Sloat, R. L. 1978. Letter to the author on the history of support for health economics research in the Public Health Service, with supporting documents.

Smith, B. L. R. 1966. *The Rand Corporation: Case Study of a Non-profit Advisory Corporation.* Cambridge, Mass.: Harvard University Press.

Somers, H. M., and Somers, A. R. 1967. *A Program for Research in Health Economics.* A background paper prepared for a conference of experts held October 29, 1965, by the Brookings Institution. Public Health Service Publication No. 947.7. Washington, D.C.: U.S. Government Printing Office.

Sydenstricker, E. 1935. The Economics of Medical Care. *Virginia Medical Monthly* 61: 574–579.

Veysey, L. R. 1965. *The Emergence of the American University.* Chicago: University of Chicago Press.

Wilbur, R. L. 1928. The Cost of Medical Care. *California and Western Medicine* 29: 1–2.

———— 1929. The Relationship of Medical Education to the Cost of Medical Care. *Journal of the American Medical Association* 92: 1410–1412.

Winch, D. 1969. *Economics and Policy: A Historical Study.* New York: Walker.

This paper was supported, in part, by Grant HS-02865, National Center for Health Services Research, HRA.

Commentary

I. S. FALK

Department of Epidemiology and Public Health,
Yale University School of Medicine

F OX BEGINS BY ANNOUNCING his focus on changes in the assumptions and perceptions of social scientists, especially economists, about "health issues"; and he runs the course from Adam Smith to current participants in the disciplines. To determine those changes he needs to consider them in various connections and over time, and thus to deal with the problems and developments with which the social scientists were confronted. With this I have no quarrel. But when in the course of his review he misreads so much of the history with which I am acquainted, and when it leads him to conclusions that I regard as indefensible extrapolations from the ground he has covered, I do quarrel.

Witness Fox's inferences and conclusions—at various points in his paper—that *reform* of medical care has been largely or mainly an exercise in futility and that it is now the more improbable because it is not compatible with the comfort of academics engaged in the teaching and research of economics and of graduate students in economics. He envisions that we now have *relativism* in our future because economists and would-be economists are more comfortable with nullity on controversial social or economic policies. And this at a time when the steeply escalating costs of medical care are exacerbating the frightening inflation in the economy, when massive governmental interventions toward containment of medical care costs is a high-level national political proposal, and when alternative designs of a national health insurance are headline news. In this scene, Fox sees the nation's course to be greatly influenced if not de-

termined by slowly evolving, philosophically impartial, economic
research in the shades of academe. Is this the world in which the rest
of us are living with respect to public policy applicable to health care
and its economics?

Neither space nor time permits me to comment on all steps to
which I would take exception in Fox's version of the history of health
and medical care in the United States, or to cite major developments in the past half-century that do not fit within his account or his
evaluations of either the perceptions of social scientists or the course
of history. But I cannot avoid comment on some of his questionable
analyses and must express my disagreement with his outlook for
what is ahead.

Fox on Chapin's Views of the Value of Life

With respect to early economic analysis applied to health issues, I
was astonished by his quotation from Chapin's 1913 paper, "The
Value of Human Life." If Fox read that paper he surely found that
this distinguished early American health officer displayed "value" in
economists' terms and that he accepted various versions of the social
and economic value of human life. Chapin was *not* arguing that the
return from the costs of more preventive medical care, etc., would be
"unrealistic," as Fox says, but that it would not be *persuasive* to
employers, taxpayers, etc., who would foresee *no monetary return to
them*. Also, Fox's passage that "Chapin warned against overconfidence in the power of medical science" is technically correct but
not in the context in which it is cited here; and so is his statement that
Chapin studied economists' arguments in order to dispute them, because he didn't.

If Fox had better familiarity with the history of public health he
would know that among Chapin's notable contributions were the
demonstrations that many long-inherited sanitary and public health
practices were ineffective and even wrongly founded, and that they
should give way to others that were likely to be better. And that
Chapin did *not* say, as Fox presents the quotation out of context,
that the effectiveness of *most* preventive measures was "by no means
certain"; he had good reason to challenge *some* that were being
proposed at the time. The real point of the Chapin paper is in his last
paragraph:

Life and health are cherished by all. It needs no argument to prove that it is good to be well and that it is wise to spend money for health. . . . Is it not enough to urge expenditures for the preservation of health because the happiness of mankind will be promoted thereby?

This, to be sure, is not an economist's argument. But then, Chapin was not an economist; he was a physician and health officer dedicated to prevention of disease and improvement of health. And he had grounds and a right to argue *persuasively* for more to be spent for health, whether or not this reduced what would be available to spend for other goods or services, or whether or not—as is often the case in public health—improvement of health increases productivity and contributes to larger global amounts being available to spend, thus reducing the competition of multiple claimants for scarce resources.

This last is my main reason for singling out Fox's remarks on Chapin: To remind economists (and historians) of the cautions to be observed when applying rules of economic analysis to health and welfare problems.

An hour with Chapin's classic report, *Sources and Modes of Infection,* first published in 1910 (Boston: Wylie), would have prevented Fox's misunderstanding.

Fox on the Committee on the Costs of Medical Care (CCMC)

Equally astonishing is Fox's review of the CCMC, beginning with his remark that "The weak connection between economics and medical care was apparent in the reports of research conducted for the Committee on the Costs of Medical Care in the early 1930s." This remark floats nearly totally in vacuo since he refers to only a few of the twenty-eight reports of the committee and to none of the many reports from its collaborating institutions.

In keeping with Fox's declared focus on social scientists, he first inspects the CCMC staff and concludes that its research, though called economics, had little in common with academic economics of the time. This, despite the fact that several held academic degrees (Ph.D.) in economics, and even taught at academic institutions.

But Fox is quite correct that the staff was not all economists and did include statisticians, public health personnel, physicians, a pharmacist, etc. Should it have been all economists, in light of the reasons that brought the CCMC into existence between 1925 and 1927—to study the characteristics and dynamics of medical care toward the objectives of making medical care more readily and more effectively available? This was not an exercise in academic economics; it was a purposeful undertaking on a comprehensive scale to search out ways for the improvement of a basic social service.

Fox appears to criticize the CCMC staff because the members

> were anything but neutral about the social value of medical care. For most of them, medical science and technology were progressive and had a benevolent influence on society. This assumption permitted them to argue that reforms that made more medical care available to more people, with costs shared more equitably between individuals and society, were in the public interest.

Apparently, this was in conflict with what he regards (in the *early* pages of his paper) as contrary to the canons of respectable economics. (I will return to this point later.) And then he delivers himself of an *obiter dictum* that would be worthy of disciples of pure mathematics: "There is no necessary connection between research and reform, particularly in the period since the 1920s." Is it graven in tablets of stone?

Fox displays a confusion about our introduction of the concepts of *need, demand,* and *effective demand* for medical care. Surely, in studies of gaps between need and receipt of medical care, criteria other than *need* (as determined by medical judgment) and *demand* (as sensed, desired, or even implored by people) were required. We used availability, accessibility, utilization, etc. Fox's confusion appears to devolve from inaccuracy possibly in reading but certainly in quoting what we said:

> The need for medical care is compounded of two constantly changing factors: the science and art of medicine on the one hand; on the other, the changing expectancy of disease. . . .

> Need and Demand—It is perhaps unnecessary to point out that the need for medical care is not necessarily the same as the demand. The demand for medical care is conditioned largely by economic factors. . . . This report makes no attempt to measure the effective demand for medical care; a study now being completed . . . will give a comprehensive picture of the present utilization of medical services. . . .

The real need for medical care is a medical not an economic concept. . . .

From some points of view, medical care can be considered as an economic commodity. . . . But medical care is not merely an economic commodity, it is also a personal service involving individual relationships between a medical practitioner and a patient. . . .

Fox incorrectly concludes that we "later blurred this point, declaring that because health care is a 'personal service' it is not entirely an 'economic commodity.' " In my opinion this statement all but inverts what we intended to say.

Concentrating attention on the CCMC's staff, Fox ignores the committee itself except for an ad hominem quotation from its chairman, Dr. Ray Lyman Wilbur. Had he considered the committee he would have found it included not only well-known physicians and dentists, public health leaders, educators, etc., but also some leading persons of the day in economics and sociology. If he had read an introductory note which appeared in each of the twenty-six staff reports, he would have known that every member of the committee (including the economists and other social scientists among them) had opportunity to review, criticize, and comment upon every such report before it was approved for publication.

Perhaps the most singular characteristic of Fox's review of CCMC is that, having focused on the committee's staff, he then virtually left Hamlet out of his play—virtually, in light of only a citation to the committee's Final Report in his list of references and a two-sentence criticism of it excerpted from a personal statement by Walton Hamilton, an economist member of the committee. It escapes me how Fox could relate that criticism to "differences between the committee's staff and the economics profession" since Hamilton was writing about excessive indulgence in compromises toward member unanimity for the *committee's* recommendations.

Perhaps Fox's neglect of the committee's Final Report reflects that he does not think—as many do—that it greatly influenced the course of subsequent developments in medical care. But do I do him an injustice by inferring he thought it of no consequence what uses the committee made of its staff's twenty-six reports, or what influence the staff studies and reports had on the committee's majority and/or minority reports?

Before leaving Fox and the CCMC, I would refer to two outgrowths from the CCMC studies to which he has apparently been insensitive and which bear importantly on post-CCMC development of medical economics:

1. The CCMC staff reports and the committee's own report portrayed convincingly that the medical care market is not the pure market of the classical economist. Here the physician as provider is also consumer of medical care; and, with nearly exclusive knowledge of medical care need, service, and value, and with nearly total control of utilization and price, he creates relationships that are not those of conventional economic theory. The long-persisting failure of economists to appreciate these nonconventional relationships bears on the failure of economists—in which Fox shares in the early pages of his paper—to apply themselves productively and constructively to the economics of health and medical care.

2. The CCMC staff studies and the committee's deliberations led not only to understanding of the finances of medical care but also to recognition of the integral relations between the financing of the costs *and* the organization for availability, accessibility, and delivery of medical care. Thus the principal rational recommendations that emerged concerned the need for both group payment *and* group practice with regional organization. And these foreshadowed the principal issues that would plague the medical care scene to this day.

Fox on the CCMC's Sequelae

Perhaps because he may not have had occasion to study most of the CCMC staff reports or the committee's Final Report, Fox fails to appreciate to what extent their sequelae have occupied health economics and health economists in the decades since the CCMC:

1. Much of the basic quantitative data for the health care industry and much of their interrelations were laid down by those CCMC reports, and—though many of the numbers have changed—the CCMC data are still many of the benchmark figures today.

2. An increasing number of medical economists have grasped the CCMC demonstration, and many of its implications, that the medical care market is not the pure or free market of classical economics and that *medical* economics therefore demands departures from some of the classical canons.

3. The finances of medical care are reflective of the composition of medical care providers, of the excessive development of specialization and the decline of the general practitioner, of the inherited structure of the industry and the inherited financing through fee-for-service.

4. The trend toward rising medical care costs to levels that price medical care beyond the reach of many persons and that become incompatible not only with the demands on spendable income but also with social policies on availability of and access to health services and medical care.

5. The need to deal with the variable and—to the individual and the family—the unbudgetable nature of medical care costs, so that the financing of medical care demands group practice as well as group payment (both of which were explicitly designed in the committee's Final Report nearly five decades ago and which have recently been rechristened "health maintenance organizations").

6. The obligations of society to strengthen the supports for the professional and technical education and training of the needed health care providers and to encourage their rational geographical distribution.

7. The opportunities for continuing studies of standards of quality of care and for continuing efforts to effect their applications.

8. In the absence of population-wide provisions for health services and medical care, the urgency to make special provisions for disadvantaged groups in the population.

9. The increasing emphasis on the need for more and better community-wide as well as personal preventive medicine, whether financed by public or private means.

Nor may Fox have appreciated that the *failure* to accept the voluntarism to which the CCMC bound its recommendations converted many of us of the CCMC and our successors to advocate medical care pluralism within the general framework of compulsory programs. And that this failure of voluntarism led quickly after the Final Report (October 1932) to the politically aborted effort to include health insurance within the Social Security Act of 1935, soon thereafter to the National Health Conference of 1938 and the Wagner Bill of 1939, and then to the long efforts mainly through the Wagner-Murray-Dingell bills to the eventual enactment of Medicare, a national health insurance for the aged, in 1965. In all of these

developments economists and other social scientists played significant roles.

Finally, I think Fox places undue emphasis on the content of
economists' journals and books and he misreads the history of the
period 1933–1979 in focusing on nonideological economic teaching
and research. He treats it as something not only apart from but also
even in conflict with economic study and research for policy formulation in both the public and the private sectors. To the contrary,
evidence abounds that many health and medical economists have
had concern for end results and have not been—and are not—content to be absorbed with only the dynamics of process. They have
been and are playing significant roles in the design as well as in the
testing of social policy for health care, alert to the particular
characteristics of its market, while many of those economists who
choose to eschew the hurly-burly of social policy design and implementation exercise their ingenuities with more esoteric concepts
and with hypothetical economic models and econometrics. Thus the
academic, as often as the applied, is—in a sense—the externality.
This may strain Fox the historian, except for his caveat that the
current scene is the preserve of the *future* historian.

Commentary

AGNES W. BREWSTER

*Health Care Economist,
Mountain View, California*

DANIEL FOX HAS PRODUCED an interesting document that attempts to explore and explain a change in the economists' views on health care, one that holds little promise for reforms in medical care delivery or financing in the near future. The early reformers who felt compulsory health insurance was inevitable and worked toward its enactment into law have, in his opinion, been replaced by academicians who make continuation of the status quo inevitable. I would not have described my role as a "reformer"; rather, I felt I was a gatherer of data that others could use to depict the reasons why revisions in our medical care delivery system were needed.

Dr. Fox dismisses the period from 1920 to circa 1950 as one in which there was no interest in the subject of health economics. One cannot help recalling that World War II might well have interrupted a great many normal interests and scientific pursuits. In this period Governor Earl Warren came close to passing a health program for California. A great number of physicians and trained researchers were involved from 1927 through 1933 in the activities of the Committee on the Costs of Medical Care; the committee's work very nearly resulted in the enactment of a program of compulsory health insurance as part of the Social Security package in 1938.

Historian Fox has made no mention of the "Clark Report" ("Health Insurance Plans in the U.S."), prepared by Dr. Dean Clark after intensive research by the Senate's Committee on Labor and

Public Welfare.[1] Both this report and the five or six volumes of *The Health Needs of the Nation* provided substantial background material demonstrating a lively interest in improving supply and understanding demand in the medical care arena. These reports showed that good medical care was affordable in the United States, given the right economic base.

My own view is that, stimulated by the work of the Committee on the Costs of Medical Care, when peace returned after World War II, economists as well as others realized the need for definitive data to back up their sense of the inherent correctness of their pressure for policy changes. They began to employ tools either not widely used before World War II or newly created during the war. I well remember explaining to the doctors in the Public Health Service that cost-benefit analysis was really just a new "buzz word" for the activities that went into preparing the department's yearly budget. How often I have wished that the techniques refined in cost-effectiveness analysis had been applied when Salk first came up with polio vaccine. We could easily have paid for universal vaccination of all the children in the country with the savings enjoyed from hospital beds emptied by the ending of this crippling disease. (Canada went ahead and did have a public program, without refined cost-benefit analysis.) Other developments that aided the economist were refinements in the cost-of-living index, to reflect medical care costs more accurately, and revisions in life tables that made calculations of the value of a man's life of toil more accurate.

Furthermore, medicine, neither very effective nor very costly in times past, began to make medical care a worthwhile, but increasingly expensive, service. When I entered this field, a day of hospital care cost less than $15.00 and physicians' charges were manageable. Knowledge of how much the nation was spending for each item of care, and the mounting infusion of public monies into this market, made statistics on the size and distribution of services and their costs increasingly necessary.

True, the concentration on studies, and more studies, and still more studies served a dual purpose: 1) research keeps funds flowing into universities to maintain their staffs of researchers; and 2) studies

---

[1]1951. Report no. 359, part I, 82nd Congress, 1st session. Washington, D.C.: Government Printing Office.

postpone making any decisions until "the facts are all in." This is a popular tactic of medical societies and, one has to admit, of Congress. As an example, data have demonstrated all too many times that fewer days of hospital care are used by the enrollment in prepaid group practice plans than under Blue Cross, so that the cost of this segment of care is less. Scitovsky's studies of the Palo Alto group practice clinic have shown that care provided by specialists has a better outcome (even if more expensive) than care by less well-trained practitioners, restoring the patient to the labor force sooner and adding to the nation's productivity and wealth.

More and more popular journals have contained articles on medical economic subjects. I still recall the day when *Business Week* was preparing to run its first definitive piece. Leonard Silk reached me from New York while I was at the hairdresser's in Washington, and we verified the text for an hour via long distance! My hunch is that laymen have had a lot of exposure to the subject and this grass-roots awareness—including labor union educational efforts and congressional airing of the problems of the aged in obtaining and paying for health care—makes the posture of academic economists less important.

Another clue to the improved chances for change lies in the sphere of professional associations. For instance, membership in the Medical Care Section of the American Public Health Association (APHA), in these same "lean years," had been growing rapidly. The section became the largest in the APHA. If one adds the Health Officers' Section to that of the Medical Care Section, and members of state affiliates as well, there would be a sizable number of people concerned with the economics of medical care and their numbers continue to expand.

While my long-continuing interest (from 1929 onwards) in prepaid group practice has been disparagingly referred to by some physicians as a "do-gooder" activity, it really stems from the patently logical economics of this form of delivery of medical care. As an oldster, who should be getting to a stage of resisting change, I still have high hopes for a system of equity and justice in medical care.

Commentary

C. Rufus Rorem

Health Care Economist (Retired),
New York City

ARLY IN THE YEAR 1928 a national Committee on the Costs of Medical Care began a study to develop recommendations for changes in the production and financing of health care for Americans. It was a period of high employment and low prices, but there was a general feeling that adequate medical services were not available to the average man, who was defined as a "person of moderate means." Six philanthropic foundations contributed a total of about one million dollars to support the project. Two others refused to help finance the venture, on the grounds that research was unnecessary and that the time had come for action.

*   *   *   *

Health care is an economic commodity in the sense that the costs of production and consumption can be, and are, measured in terms of money. But health care differs sharply from other commodities; these differences must be considered in any economic analysis.

*   *   *   *

Modern society decrees that access to health care is a human right, regardless of a person's ability to pay. This policy is defended on the principle that health is wealth, and unattended sickness or injury is a public danger and inconvenience.

Coinsurance and deductible provisions are often used to limit the amount of care to which an insured person will be entitled. The purpose is declared to be the avoidance of unnecessary care, the conservation of providers' time and resources, and the containment of total costs to beneficiaries of a health care program. Undoubtedly coinsurance and deductibles accomplish these objectives. But their enforcement constitutes the control of medicine by arithmetic rather than by professional judgment. These procedures are an offense to honest consumers, and an implied insult to the integrity of ethical practitioners and responsible management.

*　　*　　*　　*

Legislators have shown great interest in programs that would provide payments to providers when the total amounts reach catastrophic proportions that might consume a person's total wealth or drive him into bankruptcy. Such instances face about one percent of the population annually. But a person supporting a family on an annual income of $25,000 is more interested in the first $1,000 for an episode of sickness or disability than the last $100,000 that may be paid practitioners and institutions when he is broke.

Care of catastrophic or terminal illness is a proper feature of a national or state-wide program, but it should not precede or be substituted for the many services that are required in smaller amounts by more than half the population every year.

*　　*　　*　　*

Relativism in health care is a term used to characterize incremental or minor changes in some aspects of production or financing. Examples are voluntary health insurance programs, money reimbursement of interns and resident physicians at hospitals, private group practice by doctors and dentists, increased ambulatory care and emergency care at hospitals, and government programs of medical care for the aged and indigent. These changes were not developed as alternatives to complete "reform." They were alternatives to the previous status quo, compromises in a class struggle between providers and consumers of health care.

Commentary

KENNETH J. ARROW

James Bryant Conant University Professor,
Harvard University

P ROFESSOR FOX'S HISTORY of the relations between the thinking of economists and reforms in the health care system can justly be described as extraordinary in the literal sense of the term. The question whether economic analysis has any validity is not raised; indeed, the vast amount of empirical and theoretical work by able scholars is not even described. Many pages are devoted to uncomplimentary explanations of the changed attitude of economists; but what that attitude is can in no way be inferred by the most careful reader.

Fox's viewpoint is expressed in many places but never more succinctly than in his last paragraph. "[Economists] are intensely skeptical of any proposals for reform. This skepticism often irritates people outside academic disciplines who are committed to stimulating or preventing particular changes in public policy. However, relativism has made it easier for social scientists, and for economists in particular, to collaborate with physicians, health administrators, and public officials with whom they share an ideological commitment that ideology is dangerous."

In short, Fox has found a motive for economists to be careful about supporting change, namely, it upsets the applecart. Elsewhere Fox stresses not only the comfortable links with the medical and political establishment but also indoctrination into the scholarly tradition of economics, which apparently is supposed to be alien to all moral concern.

However, there seems to be a small omission here. I don't think it is mere pedantry to distinguish between the motives for research and the validity of the results, for policy as well as for pure knowledge. Economists are indeed concerned, as Fox says, about the allocation of scarce resources among competing wants. To know the effect of different pricing and insurance systems on the demand for medical services appears to me to be a very valuable piece of information to be used in any proposed reform. The sharply rising costs of medical care following on Medicaid and Medicare are a real problem for any policy. Fox nowhere asks if the many analyses and measurements have any validity or any value for health policy. One would suppose that was a far more interesting question, for health policy if not for the history of thought, than socioeconomic analyses of the motives of economists and other social scientists.

(I do not wish, even by silence, to be thought of as accepting the motivations ascribed by Fox for the "relativistic" concerns of economics. No one can doubt the importance of institutional and social pressures in the evolution of any subject, particularly those especially concerned with major social issues, whether economics or sociology. But any intellectual discipline with standards has an evolution of research in which theoretical coherence and empirical validity play a role independent of intent. The validity and social usefulness of economic analysis of health problems are to be judged by the usual canons of knowledge, not by analysis of motives. Louis Pasteur was motivated in his studies of fermentation in part by his religious beliefs that there is no spontaneous generation of life, creation having been a unique act of God; many of his contemporaries were motivated in their biological research by the desire to show that religion was a remnant of superstition and that, as Laplace put it, God is an unnecessary hypothesis; but the validity of the germ theory of disease was independent of these initiating motives.)

It is noteworthy that Fox makes no explicit reference to any studies by economists since the work of Selma Mushkin and Rashi Fein in the late 1950s (except for a brief mention of a paper of mine, whose content could not possibly be inferred by the reader). The extensive work of Victor Fuchs goes unmentioned; Martin Feldstein and his coworkers are represented only by a sneer at a passing phrase; Alain Enthoven's policy recommendations are not commented on; and the vast health insurance experiments of the Department of Health, Education, and Welfare, with ongoing analysis by

Joseph Newhouse and others, are not thought worthy of mention.

I do not have the space to write the survey and evaluation of the current work in the economics of health that was indispensable to the paper Fox should have written. Let me conclude by noting the complete fallacy of Fox's opposition between morally neutral analysis of resource allocation and a commitment to reform. I assume, of course, that reform of the medical delivery system is not desired merely for its own sake but to improve the lot of the members of society. The fact that resources devoted to medical care are secured at the expense of other uses, some of which may in fact contribute more to health than additional medical care, is in itself a factual statement. But it is a strange morality that ignores it. Further, a commitment to increase public support may still be realized in many alternative ways. Is it irrelevant whether socially committed resources go primarily for almost useless purposes, or simply to increase the incomes of physicians, or to ways that enhance the access of as many individuals as possible to medical care? These are not matters on which any amount of moral fervor will give interesting answers.

Commentary

RASHI FEIN

*Harvard University School of Public Health
and School of Medicine*

ANIEL FOX'S ARTICLE IS AN ILLUMINATING EXAMINATION of
the "history of ideas." I would not quarrel with his conclusions and, most assuredly, not with his observations that
"social scientists who work on health issues have become more
respected within their disciplines and more acceptable to physicians,
but less concerned with equity and social justice." The two
phenomena, of course, are quite related. Such is the state of
economics; such is the state of the society in which our discipline
flourishes. These are not the days of "moral philosophy" or even of
"political economy." It is not clear who, if anyone, is the American
Richard Titmuss or the next generation Edwin Witte or William
Haber, and we are a long way from 1953 when Eveline Burns could
be—and was—elected a vice-president of the American Economic
Association. *Sic transit gloria economici.*

The whys and wherefores that help explain the relative concern
with efficiency and neglect of equity by economists are many and, in
my view, include factors in addition to those discussed by Fox. What
is more important is that, in describing health economics, Fox alerts
the reader to the danger of looking to economics and economists to
provide policy prescriptions for decision making by organizations
(including government) whose concern is with equity and distributive
justice issues. At best, the economist's focus on efficiency can il-
luminate one side of the equity/efficiency trade-off, but we do little

more than that. Given the economist's status (derived, perhaps, in part from the power to manipulate data in esoteric ways and arrive at answers that appear quantitative, precise, and so very scientific), the narrow efficiency focus contributes to a distorted view of the society. Indeed, many economists (and national leaders) seem to believe that "the economy" is synonymous with "the society." It is as if the latter is entirely encompassed by the former.

Thus it is that the language of the marketplace—bottom line, marketing, sales, producer, and consumer—captivates our hospital administrators. Thus it is that the president—on grounds of efficiency—would replace elements of the Social Security system with means-tested programs in order to more effectively target expenditures. Thus the call for "technical answers, not political answers," for answers based on criteria of efficiency, not on considerations of social justice. The former presumably are precise and value free; the latter are "soft and mushy." A pity, indeed, that national health insurance was not enacted in an earlier day when technicians (and economists) had not yet been elevated above politicians. We can be thankful that we are not now engaged in a great debate concerning the validity of the concept of free public education. Technicians are not protagonists for concepts.

The problem is real and, I fear, will remain so for these are not the times when people seem ready to march under a banner that calls for redistribution. Archie Cochrane had his banner, "All effective treatment must be free"; the economist's banner is "All treatment must be effective." Those who would carry Archie's banner are defined as noneconomists, for economists are not interested in building a better society but in building better markets. Our discipline's strengths do not lie in matters of distribution. Our range of vision does not encompass equity.

Nor should we imagine that the balance between efficiency and equity is redressed by reference to human-capital theory and cost effectiveness or benefit-cost analysis. Useful as these approaches are, they do little justice to questions of distribution, "fairness," "equity," and "social justice." Moreover, their perspective (certainly given the available measurement techniques) is at variance with a broader view of man and of the role of government, say, of a department of health, education, and welfare. It is that that impelled me, over a decade ago, to argue that the title for a new series of

Brookings Institution studies should not be "The Economics of Human Resources" or "The Economics of Human Investment." I wrote a four-page memorandum whose general tone is indicated by the following brief excerpt:

> I am sure that all of us agree that many of the programs in health and in education and in welfare are undertaken—and should be undertaken—for noneconomic, humanitarian, equity, and other reasons. This is not to deny their economic function and not to deny the importance of cost-effectiveness studies and so forth. It is to suggest, however, that I, for one, do not feel comfortable with the implication that these programs are to be justified solely on their economic merits. Economic growth is important, but it isn't the only thing in life. In this connection, I remind you of some of the difficulties we had last Friday with [our visitor] on the problem of the aged and children. As I see it, he was less interested in the aged because they presumably have a lower benefit-cost ratio. But life isn't just one great big benefit-cost ratio. It ill behooves us to provide ammunition to those who think that is what economists think.

In suggesting "Studies in Social Economics," I won the battle. The war, however, was fought—and lost—in a wider arena.

What are we to make of all this? Dan Fox refers to my volume on the economics of mental illness. I tried to argue that there was an economic argument that justified expenditures on the sick. I wrote:

> Economic and budgetary problems and principles are, therefore, not the only guiding principles for the institutions that society has established for the ultimate purpose of supporting, caring for, and advancing the members of that society and the society itself.
>
> Yet, once the above qualification has been made, the fact remains that economic and budgetary considerations do have a role to play, even if it is not the sole role; the further fact remains that when resources are scarce (as they always are)—and with other, e.g., humanitarian, considerations being equal—the program that can "make an economic case for itself" has some advantage over the program that is unable to do so. ... What economic reasoning can those concerned with mental illness bring before the public?[1]

Then I presented the argument that Dan Fox cites, i.e., that the resources of the economy may be expanded by reducing illness itself.

---

[1]Fein, R. 1958. *The Economics of Mental Illness*, 127. New York: Basic Books.

In that happy world, the trade-off between efficiency and equity, between the economic and the humanitarian argument (for I, too, had adopted the terminology) is resolved. Thus, I could answer those who were troubled about the way I cast issues, that here was economics in the service of decency. How nice—some would do things because they were "socially right"; others would do things because they "paid off." Why not enlist the second group by pointing out that even if their motives were narrow, the cause of decency could still be served?

But what if the answers came out the other way? What if efficiency and social justice were in conflict? What if health care were a "poor investment," as it may be for the very old or the very young (who face a discount rate of ten percent and whose earnings are still far off), or the unemployed or low-income earners? It is in those cases that an economic efficiency orientation provides a distorted perspective. Unless the limits of economics as it is generally practiced are understood, decision makers may come to think in the same limited patterns of thought in which economists think. If we fail to warn the users about the limitations of our formulations and analyses, if we fail to distinguish between policy input and policy guidance, do we not run the risk of encouraging our politicians to look for and adopt the technicians' answers? It is important that those who define away social welfare, institutional economics, "gift relationships," whose view of economics as a social science only reflects their understanding of a university organization chart, be modest in their claims of policy relevance and expertise. If we economists fail to recognize the current limitations (and implicit values) of our discipline, there is the danger that noneconomists, dazzled by our techniques and subject to our complaints that we aren't listened to, will come to think only about the things we think about. And there is much to think about beyond efficiency.

Fox's paper is a study in intellectual history. A reading of that history should help remind health economists—and economists in general—of a day when our agenda was a richer one. Unable, or unwilling, to address questions of equity and social justice, many of us have chosen to ignore them. If the tools of our discipline are not strong enough to encompass matters of distribution and social justice, it is important that others understand that. Perhaps we can make no claim to special knowledge about the trade-off between efficiency and equity. If that is the case, however, it is important that our political leaders listen to the wishes of society, not just to the analyses of economists. The health of the nation (and of the discipline of economics) requires that those who practice public policy (and those who practice economics) understand the strength and limitations of our discipline and of our comments on policy formulation. Fox contributes to that understanding.

Commentary

ODIN W. ANDERSON

*Center for Health Administration Studies,
University of Chicago*

T HE ARTICLE BY DANIEL FOX opens up a significant line of inquiry into the sociology of knowledge, in this instance why economists were active in the health services before and shortly after the turn of the century, lost interest, and then resumed interest beginning roughly with the 1950s. It would seem, however, that the economists Fox mentions in the early period were not acting as economists but mainly as concerned citizens during the nation's so-called Progressive Era, employing a few analytical and statistical tools that economists were armed with at that time.

Insofar as I can add anything to the thoughtful article by Fox, my interpretation of economists' lack of interest is that it was not until after the cost takeoff after 1950 that the health services were particularly visible in the general and the household economy, and particularly after 1965 to economists. Far more visible was the loss of income due to disability, premature death, and unemployment in the thirties. The Social Security Act itself was mainly concerned with income transfer for the contingencies mentioned. Health insurance was placed very low on the agenda and was not considered until prominent public health and medical care enthusiasts active on the Committee on the Costs of Medical Care studies (1928–1931) brought health insurance as a problem to the attention of the Committee on Economic Security, which formulated the Social Security Act. Then, as related by Edwin E. Witte, an economist, the possibility of including compulsory health insurance raised such a storm from the American Medical Association that it was struck from the agenda so as not to jeopardize the income transfer program of the Social Security Act. My own interpretation of the influence of the American Medical Association is that its power was exaggerated. Rather, the support for compulsory health insurance at the time was so weak that opposition to it seemed powerful because it was not included in the act. National compulsory health insurance did not have broad political support. It would have ridden in on the coattails of income transfer, which, indeed, was a powerful issue, given the degree of unemployment at the time and inadequate or no old age pensions.

When economists did become interested as professionals in the discipline, Fox believes that they were not interested in equity and justice in the distribution of health services and their financing, but mainly, if not wholly, interested in adding bricks to the edifice of economic theory and knowledge. I find this difficult to accept, at least in the pure form Fox presents this case. From my own reading of the literature of economics I conclude that the economists became interested in public policy issues in the health field mainly from the standpoint of efficiency, a bigger bang for a buck, or to parallel the Pentagon metaphor for the health field, a cheaper suture in your future. The basis of the economists' conceptual and statistical arsenal is to provide analyses to make goods and services cheaper to produce, quality being held more or less constant. From the standpoint of economics, efficiency is a necessary element in equity and justice, i.e., not paying any more for goods or services than necessary. Economists did not appear to be interested in the health services until the total national expenditures reached five percent of the gross national product and approached $40 billion (1965) and were rising faster than the cost of living generally, particularly the hospital. Concern with efficiency and diminishing returns of increased expenditures on the margin became of prime and classical economic interest. Now that expenditures are exceeding $180 billion the economists are incredulous and conduct research to explain this obvious waste. Obviously, the price system must be introduced at strategic points. Supply is creating demand.

So, I would not say that economists were (or are) purely relative in their choice of research problems. They may seem to be relative in that they do not appear to attack policy problems of equity and justice frontally. In a larger frame, however, economists are operating within a broad consensus, as described by me in an article that Fox quoted. He seems to feel, however, that this framework of consensus is too broad to have any meaning in choice of research problems. There again I tend to disagree in that all health service researchers, economists included, are children of the nineteenth-century enlightenment, in which the function of government is largely that of law and order, regulation, and a minimum level of welfare for the population, within which private citizens work out their own problems more or less by both private and public means or their combination. Perhaps Fox feels that the range of economic research bearing indirectly on equity and justice in this context is so broad as to be meaningless. Maybe so, but it surely makes for rather wide-open and free-flowing political and economic dynamics. For instance, economists are generally supporting the concept of competitive options for health service delivery systems in a national health insurance framework, as do I. This concept is congenial to economists and congenial to the American economic and political style. Perhaps it will not result in equity and justice on the level that is morally necessary but, nevertheless, the suggestion is that the government buy into these options for low-income segments of the population.

On a final note, perhaps the article would have had greater depth and breadth if Fox had placed research in the health services by economists in the context of research done by medical care and public health experts, sociologists, statisticians, and political scientists. The research by medical care and public health experts laid the basis for later research by economists as the cost of health services began to impinge on the gross national product and other priorities in the body politic. Presumably only economists are concerned with money and efficiency; medical care and public health experts are concerned with need and high quality regardless of cost, and sociologists are concerned with social systems, conflict, cooperation, and accommodation (what I call who-hates-whom research) with little attention to costs. Perhaps an amalgam of the approach of the economist with other disciplines will result in research that truly describes the realities of the health services enterprise.

Commentary

HERMAN M. SOMERS

*Woodrow Wilson School of Public
and International Affairs,
Princeton University*

I AM GLAD THAT DR. FOX has provocatively raised the questions of what contributions economists have made to reform in health care and why those contributions appear meager, although I disagree with some of the assertions of fact and interpretation and on the roles he assigns to several named individuals.

I pass over his invidious use of terms like "morals," "reform," "relativism," "pluralism," etc. The notion that reform, which I take to mean change for the better, is antithetical to relativism is not supportable. The implication that pluralism is the enemy of reform is misguided. Most pluralists with whose work I am acquainted regard themselves as pragmatic reformers. Ideologues are not the only "reformers" around. And there is nothing incompatible between a concern for improved research tools and reformist objectives.

That aside, it seems to me that the appropriate question to be raised for Dr. Fox's theme is not whether economists are pushing reform in their professional writings. (If they were reform advocates they would likely be pushing in some twelve different directions anyhow.) The pertinent question is whether such literature has been relevant and useful to those interested in or responsible for reforming a financing and delivery arrangement that most people in and out of academia agree has serious faults. Are they in general contributing to better understanding of how the system works and the practical possibilities for productive change?

I agree with what I take to be Dr. Fox's view that by and large they are not. The question is why. There is no one answer; the reasons are multiple. But in this short space, there are four interrelated points that deserve particular mention in relation to Dr. Fox's paper.

1. Economists are far less empirical than is often assumed. The heavy dependence of modern economics on mathematical tools can be misleading. The mathematical models are generally built upon a frail structure of assumptions about human and institutional motivations and behavior. More often than not these assumptions, based upon classical and orthodox economic theory, are invalid for the health field—whatever validity they may have in other economic activities (although Herbert Simon, the most recent Nobel laureate in economics, long ago pointed out that classical assumptions about corporate industrial behavior also proved inaccurate when appraised by actual observation of such behavior).

Few economists have actually undertaken the grimy work of personal observation of organizational structure and behavior of hospitals, how decisions are actually made and by whom, how internal political forces operate, what motivates physicians, etc. Since the foundations of much economic inquiry are so fragile, the conclusions drawn often prove immaterial, and at times even mischievous, no matter how brilliant the superstructure may be.

2. There is little professional incentive for economists to spend much time and energy in field investigation of health care institutions. (Modern economists express small respect for so-called institutional economists.) The profession's prestigious journals do not have any large readership with any special interest in health care. Articles are judged by their technical virtuosity or application to theory. Thus academic approbation tends to create a triumph of process over purpose or ends. It thus, for example, will lend justification to the growing tendency to "prove" the self-evident because the proof may require a great deal of methodological skill—and one can always assert that the self-evident is not always what it seems. This also leads to excessive emphasis on negativism, a display of technical ingenuity in knocking down the proposals of others.

3. Standing alone, economics—like other standard academic disciplines—does not have much that is realistic to contribute to policy making in this field. In the absence of adequate consideration for ad-

ministrative feasibility, psychological motivations, institutional idiosyncrasies, organizational traditions, and sociopolitical relationships, many of the "findings" tend to deal with relative trivia or have small relevance to the large and live issues. To policy makers the exercises often appear unreal.

The problem, of course, is equally true of other academic disciplines with their artificially contrived boundaries. The term "health economics," as generally used today, is a misnomer. Probably the most influential book written by a professional economist in the past decade is Victor Fuchs's *Who Shall Live?* It was effective and useful because throughout it was animated and informed by the peculiar psychological, historical, political, and sociological factors in health care. But the system of rewards in academia does not give great weight to influencing public policy or working in interdisciplinary contexts.

4. Economics is now a discipline very different from that of the twenties and thirties. Its technical armamentarium is far more extensive and its practitioners are called upon to perform tasks for which they were not equipped earlier, tasks that often involve sheer objective measurement. A gerontologist may ask an economist to measure what the economic value of an average male life is at age fifty. Or a planner may request a study of the effect a given level of copayment has had upon the utilization of ambulatory services at a Health Maintenance Organization. The worth of such nonnormative studies should not be undervalued. There can be ample good in inquiries that do not directly lead to reform proposals.

A related aspect of that phenomenon is the fact that the earlier generations of economists selected projects presumably because of their own strong interest in the subject. They were generally not subsidized. With the coming of the era of grants and contract research, projects often became attractive to the degree of their outside support rather than the concern of the researcher. Projects are often not the intellectual invention of the researcher but a response to an inviting request for a proposal. Such undertakings are surely less likely to generate passionate demands for reform than those that originally spring from the concerns of the researcher himself. The proliferation of "health economists" in recent years is not wholly attributable to any phenomenal burst of intellectual interest in the subject matter!

However, I believe it wrong to conclude that economists care less about societal ills than other people or other scholars or that they are less concerned with moral values. In academia people generally behave as academics are expected to behave. It is interesting to note that the people in an earlier period whom Dr. Fox cites for the reform fervor in their writings were in the main not academics. At the same time, we must note that there are always exceptions to generalizations. Dr. Fox fails to give adequate recognition to that small minority of contemporary economists, and other social scientists, who have indeed contributed relevantly and usefully to health affairs.

Commentary

ELI GINZBERG

*Department of Economics,
Columbia University*

B Y WAY OF INTRODUCTION LET ME SAY that I found Dr. Daniel
Fox's article an intriguing contribution to the contemporary history of social science in the United States. I am in
substantial agreement with his basic thesis that a shift occurred from
the earlier reformers to the later methodologists, and that what
happened, what is happening, and what may happen as economists
inundate the health arena is worthy of attention. I am pleased to add
one "insider's" view of this development in the hope of providing
some additional perspective.

My direct involvement, like that of Herbert Klarman, stems
from World War II when we served respectively as director and
assistant director of the Resources Analysis Division of the Surgeon
General's Office, War Department, with responsibility for providing logistical advice on the allocation and utilization of manpower
and facility resources. As a direct consequence of this wartime experience, we served together again in 1948–1949 on the Committee
for the Future of Nursing[1] and the New York State Hospital study.[2]

Except for an occasional scholarly effort or consulting assign-
ment, I had no further involvement with the health arena until the

---

[1]The Committee for the Future of Nursing, Eli Ginzberg, chairman. 1948. *A Program
for the Nursing Profession.* New York: Macmillan.

[2]Ginzberg, E. 1949. *A Pattern for Hospital Care.* New York: Columbia University
Press.

mid-1960s. Given my interest and experience, it was inevitable that I would be drawn back into the field with the enactment of Medicare and Medicaid and the recognition of their complex implications for policy. The lack of hospitality of the medical establishment to interloping economists was revealed to me by the career experiences of Klarman, who had remained in the field throughout the fifties and early sixties. Unlike most of the recent methodologists, Klarman and I brought to the health arena intimate knowledge of its institutional structure and mechanisms, always keeping that framework in mind in setting questions or looking for answers.

When Milton Friedman was finishing his study of professional incomes in the late 1930s, proving to all who would listen that organized medicine was a monopoly using controls over supply to raise physicians' earnings, I was not impressed by the cogency of his conclusions. Clearly, the model of a competitive market could not be used to determine entrance into the profession or earnings. I was struck at the time, and still am, that existing deviations in outcomes from the competitive model do not necessarily commend a public policy of more competition as Feldstein, Enthoven, Havighurst, and many other neoconservatives are advocating.

The large infusions of money into the health arena after World War II via health insurance, hospital construction, biomedical research and educational expansion took care of the most urgent problems. The fight over National Health Insurance was lost but the "old guard" from the 1930s remained and never conceded. As a consequence, few new policy issues emerged. The Eisenhower era was not conducive to public debate over unsolved problems.

By the early sixties at the first Conference on Health Economics at the University of Michigan (1962) the title of my presentation was a warning: "Medical Economics: More Than Curves and Computers."[3] The macroeconomists and econometricians were moving to the fore and I questioned their ability to "achieve understanding of or control over the economics of health and medical planning . . . [because] of the lack of knowledge of economists concerning the structure and functioning of the relevant institutions."

---

[3]Ginzberg, E. 1964. Medical Economics: More Than Curves and Computers. In *The Economics of Health and Medical Care.* Proceedings of the Conference on the Economics of Health and Medical Care, May 10–12, 1962, University of Michigan.

I did not see any easy way to reconcile the differences in orientation between the needs of the nation for policy guidance and the growing interest of economists in using the health arena for analytical exercises and methodological refinements. When Margaret Mahoney was still at the Carnegie Corporation, I advised her to finance the postgraduate training of a limited number of able young physicians in the social sciences with the aim of preparing the best of them to serve as professors of social medicine at leading medical schools. The Clinical Scholars Program at Carnegie and the R. W. Johnson Foundation shared this objective, but not for long.

Despite the rapidly growing numbers of social scientists who are now actively engaged with various aspects of the health care arena—economists, sociologists, political scientists, and still others—I have yet to see any substantial contribution to policy guidance. The barriers to such contributions are formidable and include the following:

1. An inadequate acquaintance with the structures and operations of the key provider groups—physicians, hospitals, the Blues [Blue Cross and Blue Shield], and government bureaucrats.

2. A selection of problems to investigate that fall within a single discipline. Most policy issues, however, are interdisciplinary and, as a result, much of the research outcome is lopsided, if not irrelevant.

3. The preference of economists to work with existing data that in many cases are not suitable for reaching judgments about alternative policy decisions.

4. The preoccupation of discipline-oriented investigators with the attempt to command the respect of their confreres by pursuing methodologically sophisticated approaches even if the results turn out to be nonsensical. Witness Uwe Reinhardt's amusing illustration of the researcher who found that the optimal admission flow to a hospital was "no patients"!

5. The reluctance of many academics to make the leap from research to policy.

6. The related belief that such an extension is a violation of the canons of scholarly behavior, which, in their naive view, requires them to pursue a value-free approach. Translated, this means an alignment with the status quo.

7. The shortcomings of economics in providing useful models for the study of the health care system, since the dominant conceptualization of competitive markets, profit-seeking or even "satisfying" enterprises, improved consumer choices, substitutability, and many other analytic tools is not only irrelevant but outright misleading.

Having called attention to these obstacles that stand in the way of intellectual progress and improved policy formulation, I must quickly add that the outlook is not entirely bleak. Among the young graduate students who are currently being trained by market economists, adherents of the human-capital school, econometricians and the others who stand in the forefront of the discipline, many will not stay in academic life, writing for their colleagues and instructing their pupils in the same tradition as they were taught. A growing number will move on to pursue careers in an industry that will reach the $200 billion mark this year. Here they will live and respond to the forces in the real world, adapting their theories and tools to the problems at hand. In my view, their analyses will be more pertinent. The open question is, Will they see themselves solely as technicians, coopted by the "system," or will at least a few of them look ahead and concern themselves with ways in which both the equity and efficiency of the health care system can be enhanced?

American society still has a considerable way to go before the hordes of professionals and managers[4] transcend their occupational environment and go beyond just practicing their skills to exercise their rights of citizenship and seek to improve that environment. But that may happen, possibly faster than even optimists would anticipate.

---

[4]Ginzberg, E. 1979. The Professionalization of the U.S. Labor Force. *Scientific American* 240 (March): 48–53.

Commentary

HERBERT E. KLARMAN

Graduate School of Public Administration,
New York University

T HE NEOPHYTE DOES NOT KNOW what is the appropriate posture to assume when one's work is viewed for the first time
by a professional historian. It would be churlish to nit-pick at
details, and particularly ungracious when the historian is so kindly
disposed toward my own contributions. I have therefore decided to
speak to Dr. Fox and show him some of the minor errors of his ways,
and he has kindly agreed to listen to my anecdotes and to take cor-
rective action as he sees fit. In addition, at the editor's invitation, I
have rewritten (mostly by expanding my notes) a short presentation
on health economics research that I delivered virtually impromptu as
a member of the Committee on Health Services Research, Institute
of Medicine, in Washington, D.C., on November 6, 1977.

The following comment on Dr. Fox's paper can be—and
is—brief. It concerns largely matters of emphasis and a few of the
higher spheres of economics that a mere historian may aspire to but
obviously cannot attain.

I should prefer the word "objective" to "neutral" in describing
the later health economists' attitude toward research on policy
issues. As Dr. Fox points out, the individual economist does have
value judgments and policy commitments. He even has a bias as to
the kinds of problems he chooses to examine. However, the
economist today does try to achieve objectivity in describing the existing situation and in exploring the implications of alternative
policies, even if he is not always successful in this endeavor. I do
believe that failure to achieve objectivity in analysis is often as much
due to personal temperament and attitude toward future risk and uncertainty as to ideology.

Nor do I believe that the acceptability of one's policy views to
one's peers in the academic discipline and to physicians implies a
lesser concern for equity and social justice. The discipline of

economics requires command over its concepts, tools, and data; once these are mastered, they may be abandoned or employed selectively. As for physicians, many expect of the economist an understanding of institutional arrangements and of the pressures of clinical work. Others do, of course, expect a sharing of policy commitments. No health economist whom I know lacks concern over equity—or who gets what. The usual position is simply that the economist as economist has little or nothing useful to say about this.

It is my firm impression that both health policy issues emerging from the real world and the traditions of the economics discipline are strong influences on the conduct of research. The first attracts the interest and concern of the scholar; only the second can enable that interest to turn into acceptable professional activity. Kenneth Arrow's paper is a supreme example of how research in health care financing became academically respectable. Perhaps only John Dunlop at Harvard could have furnished the site for the outpouring of a sizable number of dissertations in health economics in the late 1960s and early 1970s and for bringing into the field an influential small army of well-trained economists who somehow also mastered the finer points of medical diagnosis and treatment, as indicated by the particular problem at hand.

I enjoyed reading Dr. Fox's excellent paper and commenting on it to him and to these readers. I have already passed it on to colleagues.

Yet I also demur, in part. Most economists appreciate both the potentialities and limitations of their discipline. To the extent that they do, and as they master the institutional arrangements of health care, they can help improve the effectiveness of care and the efficiency of care. At a minimum they help lift the level of public policy debate on health care issues and proposed solutions. Yet they all know that economic efficiency is not all, nor is maximizing the size of the gross national product the ultimate goal of economic activity. The value of health care is a matter of individual valuation, and questions concerning the equity or distribution of benefits are the core of politics. Virtually every economist understands that, on such matters, his role is that of a well-informed and articulate citizen, no more.

Health Economics and Health Economics Research

Graduate School of Public Administration,
New York University

THIS PRESENTATION IS DRAWN from my own experience and best recollection of readings and conversations. I have not done any new research. The presentation is divided into four parts, as follows:

1. Pre-1960.
2. Post-1960.
3. A reformulation by subject area.
4. A view from Washington, 1976–1977.

Pre-1960

Economists were working on health care long before there was a subdiscipline called health economics.

In the 1930s the American Medical Association (AMA) maintained a permanent Bureau of Medical Economics or Medical Economics Research. The Committee on the Costs of Medical Care (CCMC) conducted numerous surveys, studies, and analyses, off which the research community lived for a long time. Milton Friedman and Simon Kuznets at the National Bureau of Economic Research (NBER) were studying professional incomes—with much emphasis on comparisons between physicians and dentists. This proved to be highly influential in thinking by economists about medicine, and was reenforced by Friedman's own later writings and by Reuben Kessel's 1958 article on medical price discrimination as evidence of monopolistic behavior.

In the 1940s, after World War II, Seymour Harris at Harvard was studying public expenditures for health care. He saw the importance of direct payments to providers at a time when cash benefits to recipients of public assistance were still dominant.

Eli Ginzberg at Columbia was studying the economics, especially finances, of hospital care for the New York State Hill-Burton agency. He did this shortly after completing a report on nursing, which recommended a substantial shift of staffing from registered nurses to licensed practical nurses.

By then the CCMC staff had dispersed, and most moved to the Social Security Administration (SSA), where they estimated the aggregate statistics on health care expenditures, voluntary health insurance, actuarial projections of the cost of national health insurance, and conducted surveys of independent prepayment plans. The names are familiar: I. S. Falk, Louis Reed, Margaret Klem, and Agnes Brewster.

Selma Mushkin had moved to the Public Health Service (PHS) from SSA. Indeed, there was considerable staff exchange between PHS and SSA, with the Hill-Burton division of the PHS serving as a site for intramural research. This was Dorothy Rice's first job, working with Louis Reed.

In 1945 the Friedman-Kuznets book was published. It attracted much attention in the economics profession, both for its findings and for its technical sophistication in applying advanced statistical techniques to the available, scanty data.

The early 1950s saw several developments, and then activity quieted down for a while. The Brookings Institution embarked on a major, all-encompassing project in health economics. Everybody waited for the publication, and was disappointed.

In 1950 the American Economic Association (AEA), under Milton Friedman's promotion (Friedman was in charge of the program in behalf of Frank Knight, then president-elect), held its first session on medical economics. Jerome Rothenberg's paper applied the new welfare economics. A. C. Kulp of the Wharton School pointed out that health insurance is not neutral.

In 1951 the *Quarterly Journal of Economics* published what was essentially a debate on national health insurance by the Campbells and I. S. Falk. Dick Netzer also intervened.

The *Journal of Business* and the *Harvard Business Review* each published an article of mine on the economics of hospital care. The latter, addressed to a lay audience, attracted more attention.

The National Manpower Council, staffed by Eli Ginzberg, prepared a report on the professions. I drafted the chapter on physicians. The council also held a conference on allied health manpower.

In 1951 the Health Information Foundation (HIF) gave a sizable grant to Oscar Serbein of the Columbia Graduate School of Business to study health care expenditures and health insurance. Although the report was pedestrian, able staff developed.

When HIF, with pharmaceutical funds, first changed leadership, George Bugbee, the new president, hired Odin Anderson as research director. In 1953 they conducted the first nationwide survey ever of health insurance enrollment and benefits. They also continued to provide small research grants to behavioral scientists, but not to professional economists. HIF employed economists, but these never occupied leadership positions at HIF or its successor, the Center for Health Administration Studies, University of Chicago.

In government, the National Security Resources Board hired its first medical economist in 1951. The agency was dying, and outside economists were not receptive to its offers of research grants.

The Magnuson Commission (The President's Commission on the Health Needs of the Nation) performed its work in 1952. Volume 4 on economics and finances, which were generally viewed as identical, contains essays by Seymour Harris, Falk, and Harold Groves of Wisconsin, and data compilations by William Weinstein of the U. S. Department of Commerce, the site of periodic surveys of earnings in the independent professions. The Commerce Department had received completed questionnaires from approximately 50,000 M.D.s in 1949, which permitted for one time only the publication of physician earnings data for large cities. Initial attempts were also made in the statistical section of volume 4 to cross-classify health care expenditures by object (hospital care, physician services, etc.) and by source of payment (tax funds, insurance, self-pay, etc.).

SSA continued its data work in the early 1950s, but was circumspect on policy pronouncements.

As noted earlier, the later 1950s were rather quiescent.

Another AEA session in medical economics was held in 1955, sponsored by Edwin Witte of Wisconsin, then president-elect, who had been staff director for the Committee on Economic Security in 1934.

In 1954, the Hospital Council of Greater New York hired the first Harvard Ph.D. in economics, who had written a dissertation on the economics of cancer under Seymour Harris's supervision.

Post-1960

The interval 1961–1962 was a watershed period, when the newly renamed subdiscipline of health economics emerged as a visible entity. There was a conjuncture of events: Victor Fuchs, then at the Ford Foundation, proved to be highly instrumental. He was interested in HEW (Health, Education, and Welfare), and sponsored six papers in three fields, back to back between theory and empirical application. The health field got Kenneth Arrow's paper in the *American Economic Review* and my own book, *The Economics of Health,* for $1,500 each.

The first national conference on medical or health economics was organized and led by Selma Mushkin. Rashi Fein and Burton Weisbrod had just written their books on cost-benefit analysis. New people appeared at the Ann Arbor conference—Gerald Rosenthal, Anne Scitovsky, Nora Piore.

For the year 1962, SSA revised its data on health care expenditures, initiating a new systematic framework that cross-classified objects of expenditure by source of payment.

In 1962 the first economist was appointed to the Health Services Research Study Section of the National Institutes of Health. Before 1962 research grants had been awarded to Mary Lee Ingbar at Harvard and to Donald Yett, first at Ohio State and later at Washington University, St. Louis. The study section was active in health economics beyond the review of applications and the award of grants. It held an informal conference, with Richard Musgrave as chairman, and commissioned four papers by economists in its two sets of Health Services Research Papers published as supplements to the *Milbank Memorial Fund Quarterly* in 1966. The four papers were by Kenneth Boulding of Michigan; Victor Fuchs, a last-minute substitute who published his first paper in health; Paul Feldstein of Michigan; and Dale Hiestand of Columbia, who had been on Serbein's staff. Fuchs's paper pointed to his subsequent research on the influence of health care on health status, and he assembled a group of workers at NBER. Included among them were Richard

Auster and Morris Silver of City College. Irving Leveson and Michael Grossman, under Jacob Mincer and Gary Becker, completed their dissertations in health economics at Columbia and worked at the NBER.

What was most astonishing in the mid-1960s was the steady flow of dissertations from Harvard on the economics of health. Under John Dunlop and then Martin Feldstein, Gerald Rosenthal, Ralph Berry, Frank Sloan, Joseph Newhouse, Robert Evans, Paul Ginsburg, David Salkever, Louise Russell, and Jan Acton received their doctorates in economics.

The Brookings Institution sponsored occasional papers on health economics. My paper on syphilis and Thomas Schelling's on the value of human life had to do with the valuation of benefits from public expenditures.

In the year 1966–1967 the Gottschalk Commission performed a cost-effectiveness analysis of hemodialysis vs. kidney transplantation for the federal Office of Management and Budget.

Throughout the 1960s, SSA remained a leader. Dorothy Rice and her young staff made continuing refinements and improvements in the annual articles on health care expenditures and voluntary health insurance. Rice's work on the cost of illness became widely used. After Medicare was enacted, SSA paid the American Hospital Association for special surveys of audited reports of hospital finances; sponsored a temporary expansion by the Bureau of Labor Statistics of the medical care component of the Consumer Price Index (CPI); analyzed Medicare data, drawn from a dual data system that was redundant by design; and held academic seminars for its own professional staff, with papers delivered by outside professors and by grantees reporting on completed research.

Several new journals were founded—*Medical Care, Inquiry,* and *Health Services Research.* Established medical and public health journals became hospitable to articles by economists.

Toward the end of the 1960s it was time for a second nationwide conference on health economics. The Ford Foundation paid for it and The Johns Hopkins University sponsored it. The conference dealt only with empirical research and deliberately excluded policy concerns on a grand scale. A new group of young authors was sought out to deliver papers; old-timers served as discussants. Also published in the proceedings were three summaries of dissertations from Harvard, Yale, and Princeton. If one reflects on the policy issues that were under active consideration at the time, all were either covered or finally excluded only for lack of pertinent data.

There was perhaps one exception: financing. There was real concern by the committee who organized the conference that the financing issue was still ideological. However, Arrow's 1963 article did make it acceptable to write on health insurance in the professional journals. Martin Feldstein subsequently showed how the powerful tools of econometrics could be applied with ingenuity, skill, and verve to available scattered data.

A number of economists undertook research in health care financing after the Baltimore conference, focusing on the source of increase in health care expenditures. Included was some joint work by The Johns Hopkins University and SSA, which was financed by the National Center for Health Services Research (NCHSR). Through its then Committee on Publications, NCHSR sponsored monographs by Martin Feldstein on hospital care and by Victor Fuchs and Marcia Kramer on physicians' services. Karen Davis worked first at SSA as a Brookings Fellow and then at Brookings. Hers was solid work technically, yet understandable to the intelligent layman. All of this research, I believe, became influential in the subsequent policy debate.

A Reformulation by Subject Area

Interest in subject matter has changed from time to time. Such shifts are due in part to technical developments in economics; or may reflect a sense of scientific impasse on the one hand or an opportunity for scientific breakthrough on the other hand; and finally it may represent mere fad, which is not unique to this field.

In my judgment the discussion of health care financing has been lifted to an appreciably higher level of sophistication and knowledge. I say this, despite the fact that economists missed the problem of provider reimbursement after Medicare and Medicaid, because Martin Feldstein forgot to consider it in his seminal work.

Still under way is the Rand experiment on health insurance and the NCHSR-NCHS survey of consumer health care expenditures. The former was not approved by an ad hoc advisory group and was also opposed by HEW staff. The latter survey, I am glad to report, will employ an improved definition of income.

Donald Yett did good work on the economics of nursing, but took too long in publishing his monograph. Others have done good work on auxiliary health personnel, but I suspect that the recent expansion in the physician supply may have rendered the problem of substitution moot.

Under the influence of the Friedman-Kuznets work and Kessel, some economists have continued to stress the physician shortage. Eli Ginzberg always questioned it, as did Frank Dickinson of the American Medical Association (AMA), until the AMA decided after the 1964 election never again to be on the losing side of a major political battle. Gregg Lewis of Chicago questioned the Friedman-Kuznets findings on technical grounds, as did Lee Hansen of Wisconsin. Finally, so has Uwe Reinhardt of Princeton in his continuing research on physician productivity.

Economists have done good work on the economics of hospitals, which is well summarized by Sylvester Berki of Michigan. Paul Feldstein's dissertation on short-run costs stands up after fifteen years. Good work was done on long-run costs by John Carr, Paul Feldstein, Ralph Berry, Harold Cohen, Judith and Lester Lave at Carnegie-Mellon, and Martin Feldstein; and the profession had the good sense to stop research in 1970, pending improvements in data on patient mix. Robert Evans at British Columbia has picked up this line of research. I have already referred to the work on hospital expenditure increases; even before analysis, economists introduced a firm framework for classifying data, which is capable of displaying annual rates of change in an unambiguous fashion. The framework proved to be very useful and, I believe, important, if description is to point the way to analysis.

All health economists missed the effects of Medicare and Medicaid—we were wrong on use and also wrong on cost or price. It is difficult to judge whether with so many more researchers at work today the same mistakes could happen. Moreover, later work by Karen Davis has demonstrated how unequal in incidence uniform benefits can be.

Starting with Victor Fuchs, some economists have focused on health outcome, on the effectiveness of care. Few, however, succumbed to the easy temptations of Planning, Programming, and Budgeting (PPB). From emphasis on the valuation of benefits economists have moved on to problems of research design: what difference does a given program make? Under the leadership of

Selma Mushkin, the profession is now shifting from the earnings approach of valuation of benefits to the question of willingness to pay. Meanwhile the emphasis in actual research is on cost-effectiveness analysis.

Economists have been favorable toward Health Maintenance Organizations (HMOs) for the most part. Prices and marketlike incentives appeal to them. Surprisingly, economists missed the labor union opposition to the 1973 HMO Act; and they said little in advance about the high voluntary insurance premium that resulted from the broad prescribed-benefits package.

Few economists have worked in health planning. An obvious exception is the Laves' monograph on the Hill-Burton program. I attribute the neglect of health planning to lack of exposure and experience at the local level, where health services are rendered. Economists' exposure to Washington is ample, perhaps too much so. Another notable recent exception to the neglect of evaluation of actual programs in planning or associated regulation is the study by Salkever and Bice of the Certificate of Need procedure. Their study raises problems of data availability and the employment of proxies.

Continuing to be neglected is economic research in mental illness. Frank Sloan made a stab at it. Burton Weisbrod is participating in a true experimental study.

View from Washington, 1976–1977

Last year I spent a sabbatical year in Washington on leave from New York University and as a Guggenheim Fellow. NCHSR furnished a desk and secretary and imposed few responsibilities. I learned that several federal agencies now perform health economics research: the National Center for Health Services Research (NCHSR); the National Center for Health Statistics (NCHS), Division of Analysis; SSA, now Health Care Financing Administration (HCFA); Veterans Administration (VA); Council on Wage and Price Stability; Office of Technological Assessment (OTA); General Accounting Office (GAO); and the Federal Trade Commission (FTC).

The multiplicity of sites for research does not perturb me. I believe that the several agencies do keep informed of others' activities. What does worry me is the quality of the intramural research work; it could be much better. At HCFA, I think, perhaps less care is exercised today than formerly under SSA.

Most of these agencies, as well as NIH, sponsor outside research. Again, I prefer a multiplicity of funding sources. And again, I think that the agencies do really inform one another. The problem is that applicants for funds do not know who has money and where to apply.

Increasing emphasis on targeted research and contracts leads one to wonder about the payoff. Consultants' reports are long and often go unread.

There must be better ways. Martin Feldstein's and Victor Fuch's books, with reviews by Jerome Rothenberg and Kenneth Arrow, show us some of the possibilities. They were bought cheaply, at $2,500 each. Of course, Feldstein and Fuchs were being supported by large research grants at the same time. And, it is fair to add, two other volumes commissioned by the same committee did not bear fruit of equal quality.

One hears criticisms of the timeliness and responsiveness of health economics research to real-life problems. My own view of the record is that on the whole it has been good, even when not wise. Too much can be made of the latest fad; often it is an old idea with a slightly new wrinkle.

The problems of health economics research are no different from problems in other research areas, in the matter of quality assurance. The quality of research and measures for maintaining that quality are central. With patience, the application of sound research findings is virtually bound to come; it usually has in the past. The Gottschalk Committee's report is a prime example.

To improve and promote quality in research, we need good training, peer discipline, and a favorable work environment for researchers.

An earlier version of this paper was presented orally by the author, as a member of the Committee on Health Services Research, to the Institute of Medicine, Washington, D. C., on November 6, 1977.

Comment on Fox and
His Commentators

DONALD FLEMING

*Department of History,
Harvard University*

I F I MAY TURN THE TABLES on Daniel Fox by alluding to his own history, he began his career with a highly regarded biography of Simon Patten, one of the principal American antagonists of Social Darwinism in the burgeoning profession of economists at the end of the nineteenth century. In the cause of putting Spencerian laissez-faire to rout, Patten candidly advocated a whole platform of concrete social reforms, ranging from maximum hours and minimum wages to diversification of the workingman's diet and federal funding of education. In the process, Patten played a fundamental role in liberating American social workers from their Spencerian prepossessions. In a still larger context, Patten was the mentor of Rexford G. Tugwell and a tutelary spirit of the New Deal.

Fox justifiably feels that there are no Pattens bestriding the economics of health care in the 1970s, no fiery prophets of reform fanning the social conscience on this theme. Though Fox confines himself to the issue of health care, the point is of wider applicability. The only American economist who is even remotely essaying the functions of a contemporary Patten is J. K. Galbraith; and he, for better or for worse, is not the model upon whom younger economists are trying to pattern themselves.

I conclude that though by no means all economists were Pattens even in 1900, Fox is correct in perceiving a big shift between

1900 and 1980 in the posture of economists addressing themselves to urgent social problems. The difficulty comes in defining what the shift was from and what it was toward, and like many of the other commentators, I am uneasy about Fox's formula *"from reform to relativism."* I do not think that "reform" has been proscribed by the development of economics, though its relationship to economics has certainly changed from earlier perceptions of this. As for "relativism" as the position at which economists have now arrived, I regard this as a red herring pointing away from the real issue.

Many trends in economic thought have converged in the course of the twentieth century, not upon relativism, but upon something entirely different for which there does not appear to be any agreed-upon term—perhaps "antiprescriptivism" will serve; i.e., the candidly avowed incapacity of economics to prescribe the ultimate goals and underlying values of society. Antiprescriptivism is the true source of the malaise that Fox feels about contemporary economics, and the malaise is intelligible only against a backdrop of the historical developments that divested economics of its earlier claims to prescriptiveness.

Summarily put, three principal forms of prescriptiveness were commended by classical (chiefly British) economics in the century between Waterloo and Sarajevo. The earliest of these to intrench itself was the economists' secularization of the puritan ethic of thrift and self-denial, the curbing of appetites and deferral of satisfactions, as the key to economic advancement. In Malthus, this prescription modulated into an ethic of self-reliance and abstention from philanthropy. With appropriate reenforcements from Spencer and Darwin, economic and biological imperatives were seamlessly welded together in a providential concatenation. Contrary to general impressions, Darwin was at least as scathing as Spencer on the "dysgenic" effect of public health measures in enabling the unfit to survive and propagate.

The third and subtlest of the prescriptive postures associated with classical economics was rooted in the Benthamite fallacy of the interpersonal comparability of satisfactions. When this was eventually translated by Alfred Marshall into the proposition that an extra pound (sterling) will always yield less satisfaction to a man with more money than to one with less, it was available for appropriation by A. C. Pigou in the book that launched welfare economics as a separate field. Subject to considerations of productive efficiency (admittedly a big loophole), a presumption in favor of levelling incomes was inculcated by Pigou upon all rational persons. If this sat uneasily (as it certainly did) with Social Darwinian glorifications of the competitive man, it was equally prescriptive in endeavoring to compel assent to a given social posture as the inexorable instruction of science. For the classical economists, early and late, never prescribed on their own behalf. They saw themselves as elucidating the objective decrees of the God of Nature, or at any rate the God of Commerce. Accordingly, there could be no question (in their own minds) of the economists simply imposing their personal preferences, with the fallibility that attached to these.

In the period since 1900, all three forms of ethical and social prescriptiveness have been progressively banished from the main tradition of Western economics—indeed, it is arguable that an everwidening ban upon prescriptiveness has been the principal unifying theme in the development of economic thought in the last hundred years.

The first ethical prescription to go by the board was the doctrinaire commendation of self-reliance and disdain for mutual aid inferred by the Social Darwinians from Malthusian premises. It must be said that the initial revulsion from Spencerian laissez-faire around 1900 evoked in Patten and others of his generation a kind of counterprescriptiveness swinging in the opposite direction, as if natural history, properly construed, required strenuous cooperative endeavors at social amelioration. It is this particular form of hesitancy in embracing the liberation from prescriptiveness, highly characteristic of the Progressive Era and of those who carried its animus forward into the New Deal, that I suspect Fox of hankering after in his scrutiny of medical economics in the 1970s. But the spell was broken, and biologically flavored prescriptions, of whatever sort, for regulating economic behavior were extinct by the 1920s and can never be revived.

The Benthamite prescriptiveness, prolonged by Marshall and Pigou, of commending the maximization of the general welfare, to be calculated by comparing the satisfactions of the individual citizens, was knocked on the head by Pareto. When the promotion of the general welfare was reduced by Pareto to the virtual tautology of leaving nobody worse off in his own eyes and at least one person better off, no society, as Pareto himself recognized, would consent to be consistently guided by this principle. But to devise any other *theoretically* valid definition of promoting the general welfare has proved to be extremely difficult.

The last of the classical versions of prescriptiveness to receive its quietus was the most deeply sanctified of all for laymen and economists alike, the ethic of thrift and self-denial whose unchallengeable supremacy as a social good was terminated by Keynes. This was correctly intuited as an earthquake in the ethical domain as well as a revolution in economics.

The implications of these developments for the social role of economics are profound but extend far beyond this to define the general tone of the twentieth century. In some respects, as Fox points out, the authority of economists (and many other professions) has been enhanced in recent generations. We live in an age of professionalism. But perhaps as a counterweight to this, rendering the situation humanly tolerable, there is one crucial dimension in which the authority of virtually all professions and elites has been steadily reduced, and this is precisely the dimension of moral and social prescriptiveness in the realm of practical conduct.

In one sense, as has often been recognized, some social scientists of Patten's generation were endeavoring to compensate in their policy prescriptions for the slackening hold of clergymen upon the community. But the erosion of moral authority could not be permanently arrested by secularizing it, and most economists ended by divesting themselves of their ethical pretensions *as economists*. They accommodated themselves to the spirit of the age. As Kenneth Arrow would insist, this accommodation could have occurred only in harmony with technical developments in economics, and its form was decisively shaped by these. Yet it is hard to imagine any further developments in theory or technique that would lead economists as a profession to reassert their old pretensions to moral and social prescriptiveness—and harder still to imagine noneconomists agreeing to be guided by these.

The upshot, lamented by Fox and others, is a generation of economists whose services to the general public are self-perceived as analytical, instrumental, and facilitative, rather than prescriptive or peremptory, and frequently devoted to weighing the economic consequences of alternative policies in a calculatedly unimpassioned spirit—delineating the options instead of choosing incisively among them and mobilizing professionally behind the "right" solution. It is a humbler posture than many economists have aspired to in the past.

For those who are troubled by it, economists have become "mere technicians." Whether distressing or not, there is an irreducible element of truth in this perception.

Yet it is not the whole truth by any means. To make economics "value-free" is not intended to banish ethical values from the world, or even from the discourse of economists avowing social concerns and social preferences in their capacity as citizens and expounding the economic implications of these. The exorcising of prescriptiveness has been accompanied by an increasing recognition by economists of the necessity for making ultimately political choices to cope with social problems that are not only practically but theoretically insusceptible of solutions in which every rational person "ought" to concur.

Economists have not been rendered "moral eunuchs" by abating their unfounded pretensions in this regard. Any who choose are free to become moral athletes in defense of their own conception of justice, on the sole condition of acknowledging that it is theirs. To recognize that social ideals are deliberate choices embraced in the larger human context rather than dictated by economics does not automatically conduce to "relativism." An economist, or anybody else, can hold tenaciously to his chosen values in the knowledge that he did choose them. For him, they need not be "relative" or tepidly held. By the same token, it is not the possibility of "reform" that has been subverted by the development of economic thought, but merely the effort to finesse the painful issues of reform by proffering moral and social prescriptions as the ineluctable wisdom of economics. It does not follow from this that reforms in health care or anything else will prove to be politically feasible in the near future. But if not, the economists will not be to blame.

Rejoinder

DANIEL M. FOX

T HE COMMENTS ON THE VERSION OF MY PAPER circulated by the
editor stimulated me to reconsider my arguments, clarify
my prose, and add new information. Several commentators,
however, asked me to write a different paper. Odin Anderson would
like a paper on the history of research "by medical care and public
health experts, sociologists, statisticians, and political scientists."
Kenneth Arrow calls for a paper describing research in economics
and its usefulness for public policy during the past decade. Agnes
Brewster and I.S. Falk seem to want a paper that describes the influence of the Committee on the Costs of Medical Care on research and
public policy since the 1930s.

These topics are different from those I chose to explore. My
purpose was to tell the story of the tension between advocacy and
analysis in the research on health services and medical care carried
out by economists during the past century.

Four of the comments, those by Odin Anderson, Rashi Fein, Eli
Ginzberg, and Herbert Klarman, are perceptive essays by scholars
who believe they have a professional obligation to advocate as well
as to analyze. However, a few points made by Anderson and Klarman require clarification. I do not mean, as Anderson believes, that
the "framework of consensus" he described in 1966 is "too broad to
have any meaning in the choice of research problems." My point is
that a pluralist consensus embraces a broad range of political goals
and that pluralism has led some scholars to accept as justified by
science the inevitability and appropriateness of the gradual
amelioration of socioeconomic conditions.

Professor Klarman is troubled by my use of the word "neutrality" to describe economists' stance toward public policy. I agree with

him that objectivity is the goal of most contemporary economists and that "no health economist . . . lacks concern over equity." I believe, however, that neutrality is often the result of the high value professional economists accord to objectivity in research. Moreover, though economists have private opinions about "who gets what," many now avoid taking strong public positions about who ought to get what. I find curious what Klarman takes for granted: that economists are no more than "well-informed and articulate citizens" when they address "questions concerning the equity or distribution of benefits." To find out how most economists came to hold this view, rather than to assert that their opinions about equity were grounded in their professional expertise, is important.

Professors Arrow and Somers make what appear to be conflicting points. Arrow believes I have not taken the internal history of economics seriously enough. Somers, in contrast, asserts that I have been too respectful of economists' methods and professional concerns. They agree, however, that I have "uncomplimentary" (Arrow) and "invidious" (Somers) views about economists' attitudes toward public policy. My paper is about economists' perceptions of proper professional activity and the relations between events within the discipline and the society in which economists work; it is not about the validity of economic analysis. Judgments, whether invidious or laudatory, about the methods and beliefs of economists would prevent historical analysis.

Because Arrow and Somers want me to judge economics, they assume that the words I used to describe change over time are judgmental. It is not invidious to describe an intellectual stance as, for instance, pluralist. Neither is it uncomplimentary to explain that economists are influenced in their work by events in the society in which they live. Economists' perceptions are formed by their ideology and culture, that is, by external events, as well as by the internal history of the discipline.

Arrow demonstrates a point I tried to make in the paper about the attitude of contemporary economists toward advocacy. He argues that guidance for the proper allocation of resources can be obtained from economic analysis, and that to the extent the analysis is valid, the allocative guidance is good for society. Arrow, like most contemporary economists, considers it proper to advocate only what has been justified by analysis. I do not disagree with this position; but it is important to explain how economists came to hold it.

Falk and Brewster mistake the purpose of my paper in their eagerness to protect work with which they were associated from an attempt to place it in context. My paper concerns itself with the discipline of economics, in contrast to what people in other fields want to call economics or to caricature, as Falk does, as "classical economics." Moreover, much of what Falk accuses me of saying cannot be found in my text. For instance, I did not say that "reform of medical care has been largely or mainly an exercise in futility."

Falk misreads my statements about ambivalence and tension, which are normal conditions among intellectual workers, as imputations of error. Like Charles Chapin, whom he quotes at length, Falk, in this comment and elsewhere, believes that the value of investment in health services "needs no argument." Questions that I believe are open, he considers to be closed.

Donald Fleming addresses important issues in the intellectual history of economic thought. I agree with him, with two reservations. I urge that relativism—the arraying of the costs and benefits of alternative policies without the assertion of personal preferences—is the contemporary form of antiprescriptivism. More important, I am not "hankering after" either Progressivism or the New Deal. My paper describes changes in the assumptions and activities of economists over time. It is intended to be as analytical and nonjudgmental, according to the rules of historical scholarship, as the work of most contemporary economists. Moreover, I have, in other settings, demonstrated my commitment to analysis rather than to reform as the primary purpose of health services research.

Acknowledgments

T HE ESSAY WHICH IS THE OCCASION for this book was prepared at the suggestion of the Milbank Memorial Fund and published in the Fund's journal. An earlier version of the manuscript had been circulated for comment by the editor of the *Milbank Memorial Fund Quarterly/Health and Society* to a number of economists, experts in research on medical care, and an historian. When these comments were sent to me, I either modified the paper to correct or clarify matters of fact and interpretation that I had gotten wrong, ignored, or underemphasized, or incorporated new data and alternative interpretations offered by the commentators when I was persuaded of their cogency. In some instances, I added new material from my own research to clarify critical points of interpretation. My rejoinder is limited to major differences in interpretation.

Several critics were especially helpful in improving the accuracy and clarity of the essay. Herbert Klarman made an extraordinary investment of time in improving it; John Dunlop made many illuminating suggestions; I.S. Falk, though disapproving, stimulated me to re-examine and strengthen a number of important points of interpretation. David P. Willis provided constant encouragement, asked trenchant questions about my data, methods and conclusions, and set high editorial standards.

A number of other colleagues enabled the essay to be written. Gerald Rosenthal has, for more than a decade, encouraged my interest in the intellectual history of health services research. Edmund D. Pellegrino provided a model of the combination of scholarly discipline and administrative responsibility. Marvin Kuschner and J. Howard Oaks have, throughout the 1970s, provided a warm working environment and a vibrant sense of the role of moral and scientific standards in practical affairs.

Daniel M. Fox

August, 1979

Name Index

Acton, Jan, 75
Allen, William, H., 13, 40
Altmeyer, Arthur, 29
Anderson, Odin, W., 41, 83, 95
Arnstein, S. R., vii, viii
Arrow, Kenneth, 2, 26, 29, 32, 35, 41, 80, 84, 86, 89, 93, 95, 96
Auster, Richard, 85

Becker, Gary, 85
Bentham, Jeremy, 11, 19
Berki, Sylvester, 87
Berry, Ralph, 85, 87
Bice, Thomas, 88
Billings, J. S., 16, 41
Blaug, Mark, 18, 20, 36, 41
Bonner, T. N., 12, 41
Boulding, Kenneth, 1, 84
Brewster, Agnes, 29, 33, 82, 95, 97
Bugbee, George, 83
Burns, C. R., 12, 41
Burns, Eveline, 63
Burrow, J. G., 15, 23, 41

Cabot, Hugh, 23, 41
Campbell, Rita, 26
Campbell, Glen, 26
Carr, John, 87
Chadwick, Edwin, 11
Chapin, Charles, 16, 17, 41, 48, 49, 97
Christakis, A. N., vii, viii
Clark, Dean, 55
Clark, G., 10, 41
Cochrane, A. C., 64

Cohen, Harold, 87
Commons, John R., 2, 12, 12, 29
Cowen, D. L., 11, 41
Cullen, M. J., 11, 41

Darwin, Charles, 91
Davis, Karen, 86, 87
Davis, M. M., 20, 31, 41
Devine, Edward, T., 13
Dickinson, Frank G., 23, 26, 41, 87
Dorfman, J., 12, 41
Dublin, L. I., 15, 42
Dunlop, John T., viii, 13, 28, 29, 30, 32, 36, 42, 80, 85, 99

Eliot, C. W., 41
Ely, Richard T., 2, 12, 12
Emerson, Ralph Waldo, 16
Enthoven, Alain, 61, 76
Evans, Robert, 85, 87

Falk, I. S., 1, 19, 21, 23, 26, 29, 31, 42, 82, 83, 95, 97, 99
Farnam, Henry W., 13, 15, 16, 41
Fein, Rashi, 28, 31, 32, 42, 61, 84, 95
Feldstein, Martin S., viii, 27, 42, 61, 76, 85, 86, 87, 89
Feldstein, Paul, 84, 87
Fisher, Irving N., 13, 14, 15, 16, 31, 42
Fleming, Donald, 97
Fox, Daniel M., viii, 1, 2, 3, 5, 6, 11, 12, 13, 42, 47, 48, 49, 50, 51, 52, 53, 54, 55, 60, 61, 62, 63, 65, 66, 67, 68, 69, 70, 71, 72, 74, 75, 79, 90, 91, 92, 93, 99